Preventing
Mental Illness

Preventing
Mental Illness

JENNIFER NEWTON

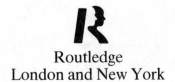

Routledge
London and New York

First published in 1988 by
Routledge & Kegan Paul Ltd

Reprinted 1989
by Routledge
11 New Fetter Lane, London EC4P 4EE
29 West 35th Street, New York, NY 10001

Set in Linotron Ehrhardt by
Input Typesetting Ltd, London
and printed in Great Britain
by T.J. Press (Padstow) Ltd, Padstow, Cornwall

British Library Cataloguing in Publication Data

Newton, Jennifer
    Preventing mental illness.
    1. Man. Mental disorders. Prevention
    I. Title
    616.87′05
Library of Congress Cataloging in Publication Data

ISBN 0-415-03963-0
ISBN 0-415-03902-9 (Pbk)

Contents

Acknowledgments

The literature which is relevant to a consideration of how best to prevent mental illnesses of all kinds is substantial. It would be impossible to cover it all in one volume. Instead, I chose to try to clarify some of the important concepts, to focus on depression and schizophrenia, and to suggest where some of the best prospects for preventive work should lie.

Many of the issues I have discussed are extremely complex. I am therefore very grateful to the following psychiatrists, psychologists and sociologists who have given me helpful comments on parts of the manuscript; Dr Douglas Bennett; Dr Jim Birley; Dr Jed Boardman; Professor George Brown; Dr Sandy Brown; Dr Tom Craig; Professor Derek Russell-Davis; Professor Philip Graham; Dr Jean Harris; Mrs Tirril Harris; Dr Colin Murray-Parkes; Dr Ian Pullen; and Dr Digby Tantam. I have also been fortunate to have the support of a steering committee at MIND (the National Association for Mental Health).

I would particularly like to thank Professor George Brown for his advice, support and encouragement throughout the project.

The research has been funded almost entirely by the King Edward's Hospital Fund for London, with a proportion of the costs for the first year supplied by the Mental Health Foundation, and I am grateful to them for their support. I would also like to thank Vicky Whitfield at MIND for her faultless typing of the manuscript.

Foreword

Preventive Psychiatry comes of age with the publication of this studious, well-balanced, and comprehensive survey of the field. Those of us who worked in the United States during the 1960s will remember the enthusiasm with which sociologists, psychologists, teachers, and psychiatrists launched project after project in the confident expectation that we would not only prevent mental illness, but improve the quality of life of all mankind. This heady optimism was promoted by Kennedy's 1963 community mental health programme which made the provision of preventive services a condition of federal funding for community health centres. Prevention was a 'buzz' word – in its name stress would be abolished, bad parents would be turned into good (and maladjusted children adjusted), counselling and citizens' advocates would be found in every street, disadvantaged groups would be welcomed by their communities, and the political symptoms which contribute to mental ill health would change.

It was fun while it lasted, but it didn't last long. The first thing to go was the money. President Johnson needed a new cause, and for a while many of the projects which had been initiated struggled on by focusing on 'urban problems', but even this source of funds was short-lived. With dwindling resources the funding bodies became more rigorous in their demands for evidence that the promise of preventive psychiatry was being fulfilled; evaluation became the order of the day, and the gallant band of idealists found themselves challenged to produce good scientific evidence for the validity of their claims. Too often that evidence was not forthcoming, and for a while the pendulum swung to the other extreme. Preventive Psychiatry was dismissed on the grounds that it had never been shown to prevent anything; academics became discouraged and turned their attention to the chemistry of the brain or the mode of action of the latest antidepressant.

In the United Kingdom the pace of change is slower than that of the States. Prevention never caught on in quite the same way as it did across the Atlantic, and similarly it never became quite so unfashionable. Although a battle has been going on for limited resources, so that all innovation is difficult, those changes that become established have tended to last.

Other English-speaking countries have taken up ideas generated in the USA and the UK and have produced their own modifications. Australia and New Zealand in particular have interesting facilities for community mental health, many of which have been developed without close links with established psychiatry. In fact, the amount of solid research and development which has taken place worldwide in the field of Preventive Psychiatry is now considerable and, despite the early disappointments, much that is worth continuing has emerged.

It is, therefore, timely for Jennifer Newton to take stock of what has been accomplished and to spell out for us the lessons that have been learned.

One lesson is that simplistic theories about human beings are seldom useful. The concepts of 'crisis', 'stress', 'social supports' and even 'mental illness' are of limited utility, and we have had to develop more subtle ways of thinking about prevention. Dr Newton has not hesitated to grasp the nettle and to devote the earlier chapters of the book to clarifying her frame of reference. The result is a subtle and penetrating work which should be read by all who value scientific inquiry into this important field. It may deter impatient fools from rushing in with half-baked schemes, but it will also provide the serious reader with the information that is needed if we are to turn Preventive Psychiatry from a castle in the clouds to a well-found scientific discipline.

Colin Murray Parkes
August 1987

1
Introduction

Preventing mental illness sounds a straightforward enough aim. First define the disorder, then identify its cause or causes, then either eradicate these causes or fortify the resilience of the individual. A moment's reflection, however, provides a hint of the enormous conceptual and operational difficulties which have dogged the efforts of those people over the last eighty years or so who have had this laudable goal. What do we mean by mental illness? Are there any identifiable causes which always or very often contribute to the development of any given disorder? If there are, do we know how to intervene to interrupt the causal process? And if we do, are the strategies the sorts of things that can be implemented by health care workers, community groups or individuals themselves?

Attempting to answer these questions takes up the following nine chapters. The difficulties involved in each of them go some way towards explaining why, in terms of practising effective preventive psychiatry, we are little further forward than eighty years ago when the 'mental hygiene' movement first began. Coincidentally, both the National Association for Mental Health here in England and its counterpart in the United States, the National Mental Health Association, have considered it timely to review the current state of knowledge on prevention. The conclusions of the National Mental Health Association are contained in their booklet published in 1986 entitled *The Prevention of Mental-Emotional Disabilities*. These two major non-governmental organisations both developed from national committees for mental hygiene which formed in the first quarter of this century, for which prevention was a central aim. It may be helpful to begin by examining the origins of this movement, and the fate of plans that have been made since that time.

Hygiene and health

In the early 1900s many psychiatrists believed that the majority of mental disorders seen by them were caused by a disturbance in the nerves or a disease of the brain. These views were tending to replace the earlier 'moral' or mental hospital movement in which the therapeutic potential of the hospital environment had been emphasised. Adolf Meyer, a Swiss psychiatrist who emigrated to America in 1892 and became a prominent figure in American psychiatry for over thirty years, attempted to reconcile the conflicting views of organic psychiatry and the declining tradition of moral treatment. He suggested a new discipline called psychobiology under which it was held that mental illnesses were a heterogeneous group of disorders whose causes stemmed from the social environment, interpersonal experiences, habit formation and personal attitudes as well as biological factors. This therefore led the way to questions about the possibility of prevention – perhaps the worst social situations could be avoided or personal behaviour changed, and some people might be prevented from developing mental illness altogether. Meyer argued in favour of acquiring good personal 'habits' and for the development of helpful community agencies, ideas which are still prevalent today (Leighton, 1982). He thought that members of disciplines relevant to psychiatry should work more closely together, especially general practitioners, neurologists and hospital psychiatrists, and that some of the essential work for preventing relapse and strengthening support systems needed to be initiated from a community rather than a hospital base. Freud's theories and the development of psychoanalysis provided further encouragement for those hoping that mental illness might be controlled or even prevented by helping people develop more healthy personalities.

Also in America in the early 1900s, a man named Clifford Beers suffered a psychotic episode and spent a number of years in mental hospitals receiving treatment. He kept careful notes of his experiences and maltreatment and developed ideas for the improvement of the care of mentally ill people. After his release he wrote *A Mind That Found Itself* (Beers, 1908), hoping to stimulate public opinion against mental hospitals. Meyer became interested in Beers's writing and influenced him to work towards establishing an organisation which would serve as an agency for the reform of mental hospitals, public education and eventually the prevention of mental illness

(Levine, 1981). Together Beers and Meyer established the Connecticut Society for Mental Hygiene in May 1908, and in New York in 1909, the National Committee for Mental Hygiene.

Some years later a similar non-governmental organisation was formed in London, called the National Council for Mental Hygiene. Clifford Beers spoke at two of their meetings in the first year, 1923. Three subcommittees were formed, and met regularly to prepare reports on the prevention and early treatment of mental disorders, on the care, after-care and treatment of the insane, and on mental deficiency and crime. The prevention committee was chaired by Sir Maurice Craig.

The National Council in London had six aims. The first two related to prevention:

(1) The improvement of the Mental Health of the Community. This involves a closer and more critical study of the social habits, industrial life and environments of the people, with a view to eradicating those factors which lead to mental ill-health and unhappiness and to educating the public in all matters which militate for and against good mental health.
(2) To study the causes underlying congenital and acquired mental disease,* with a view to its prevention. To further this, the Council will promote scientific investigation by competent workers.

Both the American and British organisations set about developing branches around the country to promote their ideals nationally. In later years, both organisations were to reflect the changes in emphasis within psychiatry by renaming themselves associations for mental *health*.

The hygiene and health movements had much in common. Both were concerned with reforming mental hospitals, with community participation and with prevention, but the latter had clear anti-medical components which increased with time. In the 1950s, mental health was increasingly emphasised, but while the earlier movement was primarily medically based, the rationale for moving away from institutional care became primarily social. Ideas relating to culture, social class, stress, social disorganisation and unhealthy roles became

* Later changed to 'defect and disorder'

prominent, and a new academic discipline came to the fore known as social psychiatry (Leighton, 1982).

Preventive proposals of the mental hygiene movement centred on child development. Good antenatal care of the pregnant mother and her unborn child was advocated, including attention to diet, exercise and prevention from infection, then regular physical and psychological checks on the child and early referral for signs of mental disorder (National Council for Mental Hygiene, 1927). The child guidance movement expanded considerably so that in America there were 617 separate agencies helping children by 1935 (Leighton, 1982).

The first child guidance clinic in England opened in London in 1927. From the beginning they have been run by multidisciplinary teams – traditionally a psychiatrist, educational psychologist and psychiatric social worker. Their aim was primarily to deal with juvenile delinquency and other kinds of difficult or neurotic behaviour in children, but it was also hoped that timely guidance would help to prevent more serious mental disturbances in adult life. The need was to unravel psychological causes that would lead to a better understanding of child development so that childhood problems could be treated and later disorder prevented (Sampson, 1980).

In the beginning the psychiatrically sick child was the central focus, but staff liaised closely with schools so that a wide range of educational problems were also picked up. This considerably increased the potential client group. However, one of the long-standing problems of child guidance clinics has been that they have often not been very successful in gaining the cooperation of parents to enable treatment programmes to be carried out. A large proportion of families referred to clinics fail to keep a second or subsequent appointment (e.g. Cartwright, 1974).

Population surveys have revealed substantial numbers of children with behavioural, emotional and educational difficulties. Intensive individual therapy can only hope to reach a very small proportion of these. Any evaluation of the success of child guidance in reducing the overall prevalence of childhood disorder would inevitably reveal the service to be a failure. They simply see far too few children to make any impact on the problem. Not surprisingly, Sampson (1980) reports that they have not succeeded in reducing delinquency, nor have adult neuroses been prevented or even made more predictable. Furthermore, early referral for difficult behaviour has been at the centre of its preventive method, yet the peak age for first referrals continues to stand at about 9 years (Sampson, 1980).

As a specialist service, child guidance clinics have had to select those children to whom they will offer individual help and find other ways of reaching the bulk of the population of disturbed children. But criteria for selecting the most handicapped children have not been clearly formulated, and priorities for action have not been evaluated. However, the movement must be credited with pioneering a number of innovative approaches. They developed methods of remedial education which have since been taken back into the school system, and art therapy which is also now more widely used. Behaviour modification has become an increasingly popular treatment in recent years, and in teaching parents how to respond to problem behaviours in their children the method may be argued to be preventive of future difficulties for both child and parent.

In later years, however, the disadvantages became apparent of a preventive strategy which required highly specialised help for individual children, and earlier and earlier intervention in the natural history of their disorders. In the 1950s Gerald Caplan, a child psychiatrist trained under John Bowlby in London, put together an alternative model, published in his highly influential book *Principles of Preventive Psychiatry* (Caplan, 1964). After the Second World War he had gone to live in Israel where he established a child guidance clinic and began to build a programme of preventive child psychiatry (Caplan-Moskovich, 1982). However, finding that many problems in children were already well established, his interest turned to pregnant women. He looked for factors that were predictive of possible later disturbance in mother-child relationships. But then, recognising that mothers were influenced in their relationships with their newborn babies by their own childhood years, and that there was no limit to how far back the aetiology could be traced, he became disillusioned with this approach. With limited resources, the numbers who could be helped were also very limited. He began to develop a new model which did not involve taking children out of their natural setting for specialised help, but instead trained the adults caring for them in the best ways of helping children with special needs. He began training other health workers, pediatricians and nurses, to become more aware of the mental health aspects of their daily work. Also at about this time, he met Erich Lindemann who was working along similar lines, offering consultation to clergymen, teachers, doctors and other 'caretakers' in Boston to enable them to help their clients adjust to crises in their lives. Caplan was impressed by Lindemann's work, and following his move to the Harvard School of Public Health, also in Boston, began to reconceptualise prevention along public health lines, defining primary, secondary and tertiary prevention (Caplan–Moskovich, 1982).

Crises became the focal point of Caplan's model, since at such times people were vulnerable to disorder, but also highly receptive to outside help. Studies of how people adapt to particular crises were expected to facilitate the development of methods of anticipatory guidance and preventive intervention. With this knowledge, he hoped that community mental health workers would be able to identify people facing natural but stressful transitions and increase their resistance to mental disorder by improving their adaptive capabilities ('primary' prevention). He also advocated vigilance for people showing the earliest signs of mental illness so that they could be referred for treatment ('secondary' prevention), and sought to develop methods of reducing the social handicapping consequences of mental disorder ('tertiary' prevention). Crisis intervention and mental health consultation were the central elements of his public health model. His lectures and publications had some influence on the shaping of the legislation for the development of community mental health centres throughout the United States during the early 1960s (Caplan-Moskovich, 1982).

But although some improvements in the form and delivery of treatment services have materialised, less progress has been made with regard to prevention. And many of the changes which have taken place in the last hundred years of psychiatry, in both preventive and therapeutic practice, have been generated from unrealistically optimistic expectations. Recommendations and generalisations from new ideas have often gone well beyond what had been reasonably established in research terms. Furthermore, it is perhaps only in the last few years that research in social psychiatry has begun to show the necessary sophistication and confidence to tackle the complex issues involved in prevention. Disappointing results have then contributed to the rejection of innovative schemes, and the theories on which they were based assumed to be faulty. Leighton (1982) describes several telling instances of this process of 'bloom' and 'blight', including the rise and fall of the belief in the therapeutic potential of mental hospitals.

Neither child guidance clinics nor community mental health centres have lived up to the hopes many of their pioneers held for their preventive potential. There was a period of optimism in the early 1960s when an atmosphere of social awareness prevailed and society itself was frequently identified as the source of evil. Prevention was therefore thought to be eminently feasible. Social activists reacted against war, poverty, pollution, technology, bureaucracy, the nuclear threat and 'the establishment', including traditional psychiatry. Society was sometimes seen as the creator of mental illness through defining people as sick, thereby forcing them into a 'sick role'.

But by the mid-1960s disillusionment was already rife. Only about 500 of the projected 2,000 community mental health centres throughout the US were completed (Leighton, 1982). Mental health workers were unable to agree on what they meant by mental health, or on what was the best way of achieving whatever it was. Awareness had grown on the size of the population with various 'mental health' problems and doubts were raised about feasibility and costs. These doubts were strongest about the ideas of prevention and promoting 'positive mental health'. 'The goal of providing services for everyone with a psychological or social need began to seem more and more like trying to drink the ocean' (Leighton, 1982, p. 72).

These problems almost certainly fuelled the scepticism of some psychiatrists towards prevention. However, in the 1970s, significant advances were made in the research on social, psychological and neurophysiological factors in mental illness. The sophistication of research methodology and standardisation of measurement also markedly improved. This attention to method at the same time brought new credibility and scepticism to social investigations. The results of some careful studies detailing links between social, psychological and psychiatric conditions had to be taken seriously. However, a disturbingly large proportion of the research, particularly that evaluating intervention programmes, has been of poor quality. In the 1980s, enthusiasm for deinstitutionalising psychiatry and developing preventive approaches continues. In North America, preventive aspirations have reached a much more advanced stage along the road between thinking and planning and doing and spending. The Mental Health Systems Act passed by the US Congress in October 1980 authorised a total of $21 million for the three fiscal years ending 30 September 1984 for preventive mental health projects, and required the director of NIMH to designate an administrative unit for overseeing programmes in prevention (Levine, 1981, p. 199). And Westchester County, New York, has a prevention programme which incorporates parenting education for low-income mothers, supportive schemes for families where the mother has been jailed, where there is a disabled baby, or where there has been an unexpected death, and an educational scheme to promote social problem-solving skill teaching in schools (Aronowitz, 1982). But a counterbalancing section of psychiatry has inevitably reacted to the overoptimism of some mental health proponents with extreme scepticism. This may prove to be helpful if it leads to caution and restraint of poorly founded overenthusiastic plans, but not if it becomes an argument against doing anything.

Barriers and incentives to preventive practice

A number of factors other than a lack of understanding about *how* to intervene have contributed to the slow progress of preventive psychiatry. Some of the issues are general ones which have affected policies for the care, as much as for the prevention, of mental illnesses. To begin with, there is the vagueness of terminology. Among the general public, the term mental illness is used to refer to nearly any state which involves a high degree of personal misery or behaviour that troubles other people. It may be used to denote disorders which are severe or mild, chronic or transitory, common or rare, or of genetic or social origins. Mental health can simply imply an absence of illness, or can mean some nebulous attractive state in which a person might be described as thriving. But at what point do we just exist and by what do we recognise someone who is thriving? Leighton (1982, p. 7) argues that use of the term mental illness has encouraged generalisation and oversimplification. This

> makes thinking and communication seem easier, but it
> misrepresents reality, creates errors in judgments, and distorts
> the transmission of information. In consequence,
> conceptualisation, planning, provision of services, practice, the
> conduct of research, and public discussion about the state of the
> field all suffer.

And of course prevention usually means stopping something from happening. But this could include not only preventing healthy people getting ill, but preventing people showing the first signs of illness from getting more seriously ill, and preventing ill people from being incapacitated by their symptoms. If we were to take Caplan's definitions of prevention, we would find that we should indeed include all of these (i.e. primary, secondary and tertiary prevention, Caplan, 1964). Clearly, having such wide conceptual boundaries to our terminology will not help us to plan services or research, or educate the public.

A second problem has been the separate developments of theory and practice, which has led to a poor use of available knowledge and inappropriate expectations for intervention. Research and theory on the origins of psychiatric disorders tend to come from workers in academic institutions who may not become involved in the translation of ideas into services or testing their ideas in experimental intervention trials. People who set up new projects are invariably practitioners responding to a need they perceive, to which they must respond in the way that seems most appropriate to them. They may be largely ignorant of research and theory and they may not consider (or have the time and resources to consider) evaluating the extent to which their service achieves their aims. Valuable opportunities for adding to knowledge are therefore wasted and worthy-seeming schemes may continue because they feel right. Alternatively, guardians of the public purse may crudely evaluate success in some inappropriate fashion that might suggest the money to be a poor investment, and the project abandoned without undergoing the scrutiny which might explain why it was not succeeding (if it was not), and how it might be redesigned to achieve the aims it was set up to meet.

Of course, evaluation of services and experimental projects is not a straightforward process. Doll (1983) describes some of the difficulties. Large numbers of people need to be involved. But they are unlikely to cooperate unless convinced of the benefits of the scheme. If convincing evidence exists that it is likely to be helpful, then there are ethical problems about withholding the measure from the comparison group. There is also the time and expense involved in waiting to discover if an illness has been prevented and the problems of controlling other important variables affecting people's health in the meantime. Programmes intended to prevent mental illness may pose particularly daunting methodological problems because of the necessarily complex and varied behaviour that is likely to be the basis of the intervention, and the need to consider the meanings of actions taken in the context of the lives of the people concerned. Judgments about the cost compared to the benefits of a service can also be perplexing. The measures may have far-reaching social effects, but if expensive, it could be that it would be cheaper to wait for the people to get ill and then spend the resources on clinical care and treatment. The perception of costs and benefits involves as much subjective judgment as objective quantification – perhaps, for instance, in assessing the value of preventing depression, which often remains undetected in the community, compared to florid psychotic behaviour that does not.

Public policy has tended to be influenced more by enthusiasm than evaluated information, and information has been generalised to problems it was never meant to solve (Levine, 1981; Leighton, 1982). And the intensity of the desire of enthusiastic workers to *do* something has tended to result in too many goals and too few priorities. The underlying belief is often that by sheer force of effort the problems can be overcome. Given sufficient money, trained personnel and resources, every problem could be solved (Leighton, 1982). Furthermore, policy makers often need to be *seen* to be taking action. Buildings are one form of proof. Nearly a century ago the building of mental hospitals out-ran the speed at which they could be staffed and run satisfactorily. The same thing happened with community mental health centres in the US several decades later. Centres had to be built while the money was available and to provide the tangible evidence that the Congress was doing something. But less money was available for staff, no time was allowed for trying pilot programmes and there was no clear idea on *how* the programme should operate (Chu and Trotter, 1974). Yet as Chu and Trotter point out, unlike general medicine, psychiatry does not need a great deal of technical paraphernalia or impressive buildings. Mental patients need a host of other things before new buildings.

Some of these problems undoubtedly contributed to the decline of the mental hygiene movement. Beers and Meyer, the two leading proponents of mental hygiene, had conflicting approaches. While Meyer constantly tried to ensure that psychobiology was studied as a scientific discipline and practical experimental services based on scientific information, developed piece by piece, Beers was much more of a crusader who wanted to organise state societies, distribute educational propaganda and *do* things on a wide scale. People began to practise more than they knew, priorities were not drawn out, and the heterogeneity of the disorders they were tackling was not appreciated.

The general shift in the climate of opinion in psychiatry towards care in the community has kept hopes high that services will be developed which are relevant to prevention as well as treatment. There has been a steady decline in in-patient levels since the mid-1950s, both in America and Great Britain. Although this coincided with the development of drugs to treat mental illnesses, certain pioneering hospitals had begun reducing in-patient levels well before the introduction of the new drugs. One consequence of the drugs was probably that they helped to change attitudes of medical and nursing staff about the feasibility of discharge (Wing and Brown, 1970). Whatever the reason for the changes, the need for community-based psychiatric services inevitably substantially increased (Levine, 1981).

Furthermore, the two world wars had given psychiatrists important insights into the nature and treatment of 'stress'. Early treatment, as near as possible to the site of the 'injury', and a rapid return to duty were found to be the most effective ways of helping soldiers to overcome psychiatric disturbance related to stress in battle. This also fuelled initiatives to site psychiatric care in the community, at least in general hospitals providing out-patient facilities, so that people experiencing stress and showing signs that they were unable to cope could be identified and treated at the earliest possible stage of developing disorder. Previously in Britain (before the 1930 Mental Treatment Act), treatment had usually only been available when mental illnesses had progressed to such a degree that certification led to compulsory admission to a mental hospital. The new moves envisaged voluntary treatment. The Maudsley Hospital in London was one of the first hospitals to take 'voluntary boarders' after the First World War.

Finally, there is the issue of motivation. Clinicians are trained to respond to clinical problems and invariably gain satisfaction from doing their best to make ill people well. Where a problem is not already manifest, there is not much satisfaction to be derived from developing anticipatory actions to prevent something that in any case might not occur. And there is no feedback to reward the practitioner for his efforts as there is when an ill person recovers, either from seeing his own success or from the appraisal of success by others. While the value of cures for distressing and life-threatening illnesses are apparent to everyone, what person stops to think about the illnesses they have avoided? Inevitably many services with preventive aims, but employing professionals trained to deal with dysfunction, quickly revert to a form of treatment. This has happened within child guidance and with methods of 'crisis intervention' operated by some hospitals (see chapter 9).

However, a fascinating illustration of what can be achieved when the circumstances exist to create the motivation for preventive psychiatry was provided by the two world wars. The need for healthy manpower was acute and it soon became apparent that the largest cause of medical discharge among military personnel was mental illness. About 118,000 men and women were discharged from the three British services for psychiatric reasons between September 1939 and June 1944 (Ahrenfeldt, 1958). In his stimulating account of the use of psychiatry in the British Army in the Second World War, Ahrenfeldt argues that this knowledge brought about the effective use of epidemiology to prevent mental illness and inefficiency.

A number of lessons were learned. High morale, maintained through skilled leadership, good discipline and adequate training, was found to reduce psychiatric problems. Even more important, however, was that the abilities and aptitudes of men were appropriately matched to the tasks demanded of them. A disproportionate number of men of limited intelligence fighting at the front as part of the infantry suffered psychiatric breakdown, as did men of high intelligence assigned for general labouring duties in the Pioneer Corps. Part-way through the war psychiatrists were allowed to recommend for transfer to employment of a special nature men who were working in jobs for which they were temperamentally unsuitable. 'This procedure resulted in a great diminution in the numbers of cases admitted to hospital because of a psychiatric breakdown and was a notable achievement in vocational selection and psychiatric prophylaxis' (Ahrenfeldt, 1958, p. 19). Eventually the importance of psychiatric advice to avoid misplacements arising in the first place was realised, and by 1942 all intakes with particularly poor selection test scores were referred for psychiatric opinion. Men considered incapable of assimilating advanced military training and who, if sent to the front line, were likely to be particularly susceptible to psychiatric disorder were recruited instead into the Pioneer Corps for unskilled duties.

The same principle of matching capabilities to demand was also extended to the rehabilitation of men who had already had a neurotic breakdown for which they had received treatment in a mental hospital. Instead of recommending the man either for a medical discharge or a return to service with the unit from whence he came, psychiatrists suggested that they be assessed for the work to which they were most suited and placed accordingly. The procedure was known as the 'Annexure' scheme and was instituted largely on the advice of Professor Aubrey Lewis. A follow-up of men rehabilitated in this way showed that 60 per cent were retained by the army, and five sixths of these had adjusted adequately and were giving satisfactory service. A return to their previous units would almost certainly have resulted in a high rate of relapse (Ahrenfeldt, 1958).

A further example of constructive preventive efforts occurred as the war came to an end, and prisoners of war were repatriated. The prevailing attitudes must have given clear recognition to the debt owed by the country to their defenders, so that there was considerable commitment towards helping returning prisoners. Following a period of extreme elation which masked any psychiatric difficulties, these men were found to have some degree of emotional instability and to be highly vulnerable to psychiatric breakdown. Civil resettlement units (CRUs) were established to cater for all ex-prisoners who wished to attend. Although the evidence as to their effectiveness is lacking, they were clearly intended to be a preventive service. After three or four weeks with their family, the ex-prisoners of war were offered a stay of a few weeks or months at a nearby CRU. The centres provided an opportunity to rest and recuperate, to learn about post-war civil life, to get specialist advice and to rediscover their previous work skills or acquire new skills. The average stay was about five weeks and ex-prisoners were assisted in their efforts to reintegrate into the civilian community and especially their home environment. They were given vocational guidance and help in finding work. Furthermore, their families were offered advice on how best to respond towards and support their returning kin.

This can be contrasted with the lack of similar help given to US veterans of the Vietnam War where the political atmosphere on their return was the very opposite. Far from being welcomed back as heroes, they were not infrequently reviled for their military acts and seen as an embarrassment to the nation. Without rehabilitative assistance, many hundreds retreated to live isolated lives in remote forests, unable to cope with their guilt, aggression and fear, and incapable of reintegrating into society. Many thousands of Vietnam veterans have committed suicide (Salmon, 1985).

The need for a preventive psychiatric service during the Second World War had one other important consequence. The effectiveness of preventive strategies had to be demonstrated, particularly when they conflicted with intended military use of manpower. Psychiatrists were held accountable as they have never been before or since (although recent developments in the funding of medical insurance in the United States may bring about a similar climate). But the numbers of men involved, the fact that they were a captive and representative experimental sample, and the speed with which a breakdown could be brought about in vulnerable men due to the highly stressful circumstances of warfare meant that evaluative information could fairly easily be gained. Among men recommended for the Pioneer Corps, for instance, comparisons could be made between those placed in the Pioneers with those allowed to procede to normal infantry training. Differences in adjustment problems and rate of psychiatric breakdown illustrated the wisdom of the recommendations. The knowledge gained by military psychiatrists may now seem almost humiliatingly simple. Yet it is not clear that it has been fully utilised in civilian life. Certainly, the political circumstances to bring mental health issues to such a priority have not existed since.

2
Prevalence and distribution of mental illness

Mental illness is more prevalent than most people realise. The DHSS (1983) gives estimated resident patients in England in 1978 (in mental illness hospitals and units) as 79,165, representing a rate of 171 per 100,000 population. At this time, 26 per cent of all hospital beds were occupied by patients with mental illness, and this proportion held in 1980 (DHSS 1982). General practitioners refer only some one in twenty of the patients they diagnose as 'psychiatric' to the psychiatric services (Shepherd *et al.*, 1966), and psychiatrists treat three out of four of their patients on an out-patient basis (Goldberg and Huxley, 1980). This means that counting in-patients gives a gross underestimation of the prevalence of disorder.

Of course, there are differences between the kinds of illnesses which are treated in hospital and those treated by the general practitioner and, on the whole, the former are more severe. Shepherd and his colleagues (1966) quote a figure of 72 per cent of all psychiatric in-patients in England and Wales as suffering from 'psychoses' (disorders like manic depression and schizophrenia), 25 per cent of Maudsley Hospital out-patients, and only 4 per cent of a general practice sample. The trend was the reverse with regard to 'neuroses' (disorders like depression and anxiety), these constituting only 18 per cent of in-patients, 44 per cent of out-patients, and 63 per cent of the GP sample. Such figures, of course, raise questions about definition, and what is included under the umbrella term of mental illness.

Most mental health workers, and perhaps even some workers among anti-psychiatry groups who argue against labelling people with any psychiatric symptoms 'ill', agree that schizophrenia is an illness. And in fact the social implications of florid psychotic symptoms are such that few people with an acute illness will survive long outside a treatment setting. This is quite unlike the situation for depression for which relatively few people are referred for specialist help, and where some will not even consult their general practitioner or be recognised as depressed if they do (Goldberg and Huxley, 1980). Compared to schizophrenia, the symptoms of depression tend to have a more ordinary quality. And the number and severity of symptoms have a more continuous distribution with no point at which there is a clear-cut change in the quality of symptoms. To decide which people have sufficient numbers of symptoms and of sufficient severity to warrant a description as mentally ill therefore inevitably means making arbitrary assumptions about what is a 'normal' response to adversity and what is not.

In considering prospects for prevention it is to some extent irrelevant what the problems are called. The aim is to prevent them. But for research on causation and evaluation of the effectiveness of intervention it is necessary to count the 'ill' and therefore to define illness. The distribution of mental disorder in the population can only be studied if generally acceptable and reliable means exist to decide who is and who is not mentally ill.

Such studies, generally called epidemiological enquiries, have many important administrative uses. They can be helpful for forecasting resources needed (beds, staff), and to inform on likely demand in both medical and social terms (age, sex, ethnic background, place of residence and so on). But their more scientific value is in providing clues to the prevention and treatment of mental illness.

The epidemiologist tries to find out which portions of the population are at greatest risk of becoming mentally ill, which recover quickly if they do become ill, and which are likely to relapse after a temporary remission. By noting who is at high risk, the epidemiologist gets clues as to the possible causes of the occurrence of psychiatric disorder and its course. He then proceeds to test these possible causes by careful statistical studies, and when they are successful, he engages in experimental epidemiology – changing the environmental factors that he thinks may cause mental disorder to show whether the plausible cause is a true cause. The final proof is that modifying that cause changes the rate of the disorder. Of course, the probable causes identified may not always be amenable to manipulation by the researcher, or government policy, and so cannot be proved.

However, it is the psychiatric epidemiologist's hope that he will discover some link in the causal chain that *can* be broken.
(Robins, 1978, p. 697)

Before turning to what epidemiological studies have revealed in terms of prevalence and distribution of mental illness, a brief outline is needed about the troublesome problem of distinguishing between 'cases', 'borderline cases' and 'non-cases' of mental illness.

Defining mental illness

What any society understands by psychiatric illness is clearly greatly influenced by the diagnostic practices of psychiatrists. However, the psychiatrist plays little part in determining which people present themselves for his advice, but in attributing a diagnosis to most of them, he or she is merely confirming the label of mental illness already rendered by others. Those referring clients for specialist treatment are therefore playing a key role in defining mental illness (Goldberg and Huxley, 1980).

But it is now clear that general practitioners vary considerably in their diagnoses of psychiatric disorder. Shepherd and his colleagues (1966) found a ninefold difference in the rate of psychiatric disorder reported by eighty London doctors. Moreover, such judgments may take into account more than psychological and physical symptoms. Hoeper and his colleagues (1984), for instance, found GPs to be swayed in their judgments by characteristics such as low income or poor education, and particularly by a previous history of disorder.

For research purposes, methods have obviously had to be found to deal with such potential variability in diagnostic practice. A number of standardised psychiatric interviews have therefore been developed which provide guidelines for interviewers that are clear enough to eradicate many of the differences between them in definition of symptoms, threshold at which symptoms are judged to be present, and techniques in eliciting symptoms. Such standardised instruments derive their definitions of disorder from the symptoms exhibited by patients seen by psychiatrists, and supply questions which can be used outside the psychiatrist's consulting room to assess the presence of such symptoms. In this way the presence of comparable disorders can be assessed in the general population, among people who have not sought psychiatric care.

For instance, the Present State Examination (PSE) is a 40-item research instrument which provides detailed guidelines about its use. Once the presence or not of the symptoms has been established, there are two computer programmes, the Index of Definition and CATEGO, to classify persons in terms of their patterns of symptoms (Wing *et al.*, 1974; Wing and Sturt, 1978). The Index of Definition (ID) provides eight levels of confidence that sufficient key symptoms are present to allow an approximate classification by the CATEGO programme into one of the functional categories of the International Classification of Diseases. The 'threshold' level five has been taken as the 'cut-off' point in many research studies as corresponding most closely to global judgments by psychiatrists that a disorder is present (Wing, 1980). Levels six to eight are allocated on the basis of increasingly detailed evidence that a psychiatric disorder of clinical significance is present.

The PSE–ID–CATEGO system was developed in London and has been used as the basis of a number of World Health Organisation sponsored research investigations. There is a somewhat similar system and equally well known which has been developed in America, called the Schedule for Affective Disorders and Schizophrenia (SADS), used with the Research Diagnostic Criteria (RDC) (Spitzer *et al.*, 1978).

However, the standardised psychiatric interviews are rather elaborate and time-consuming for use in large community surveys. This has led to the development of several kinds of screening questionnaires for the respondents to complete themselves, which provide a quick estimation of the likelihood that an individual has a definite disorder. The General Health Questionnaire (GHQ) can be used, for instance, to screen for probable 'cases' among patients attending GP surgeries (Goldberg, 1972). Probable cases on the GHQ can then be re-interviewed using the PSE-ID-CATEGO system if further information is needed. Other standardised psychiatric questionnaires have been developed elsewhere but are less widely used (see Goldberg, 1985).

Such standardised instruments enable research workers who may have differing perspectives on mental illness to arrive at similar diagnoses. The screening tools enable similar, although cruder, judgments to be made from self-rated questionnaires. But both screening questionnaires and standardised psychiatric interviews produce a distribution of disorders with no obvious division between 'cases' and 'non-cases', so that the choice of threshold as in the ID system is essentially an *arbitrary* one. Cases are not entities any more than are the illnesses from which patients suffer, and 'caseness' cannot be defined *in vacuo*. 'The division of subjects into cases and non-cases is a classification, and like all classifications it is man-made and not in nature. It is a concept created for a purpose and is useful only in so far as it serves that purpose' (Copeland, 1981, p. 10).

The cut-off between what is considered normal distress or behaviour and mental illness could not only be drawn at a different point along the continuum between health and severe illness, but could also exclude or include different types of symptoms. Homosexuality, for instance, has previously sometimes been included as a symptom of mental illness. And some systems, such as the PSE, currently do not record alcoholism, organic states or personality disorders as psychiatric illnesses. However, barring any excluded categories, the symptoms measured by current standardised research tools fairly accurately discriminate between patients seen by specialist psychiatric in-patient services, out-patients, general practice patients, and random samples of the general population and so concur with our present operational definitions of mental illness (Wing *et al.*, 1978). And these standardised measures provide a method of determining who is 'ill', who is moderately or mildly disturbed and who is relatively symptom-free. Without this ability, our efforts to conduct research would be gravely hampered; and without the means to count the 'ill', we would be handicapped in our ability to plan services, evaluate the success of treatment and rehabilitation, or to assess the effectiveness of preventive strategies.

Prevalence of mental illness

Almost all people with schizophrenia in the United Kingdom are probably in touch, sooner or later, with hospital services. Hospital statistics can therefore provide valuable information on the prevalence of this disorder. J. E. Cooper (1979) summarises the findings from fifteen surveys in twelve countries and reports a prevalence of between 1.5 and 4.2 cases of schizophrenia per 1,000 population during any one-year period. The lifetime risk of schizophrenia is invariably found to be less than 1 per cent (B. Cooper, 1978).

For most categories of mental illness, however, prevalence rates would be greatly underestimated if hospital statistics were used as the only source. Rawnsley has illustrated the different figures which could be obtained in the rate of affective disorder in England and Wales. Prevalence rates derived from in-patient hospital statistics were less than one-fifth of those derived by combining figures from out-patient and other specialist medical facilities, and less than one-tenth of those taken from studies in general practice (Rawnsley, 1968). A true picture of the prevalence of psychiatric disorder in the population can only be derived from surveys which assess the psychiatric state of a random sample of the general population, irrespective of whether the individuals are receiving treatment.

The first community surveys were conducted before standardised tools to assess psychiatric 'caseness' had been developed. The Second World War had increased public awareness about the prevalence of psychiatric disorder, and this was reflected in America by the creation of the National Institute of Mental Health in 1946 and the undertaking of a number of a community surveys of mental health. An often quoted example is the Midtown Manhattan Study (Strole et al., 1963; Langner and Michael, 1963). This project was initiated in 1952 by Dr T. A. C. Rennie to investigate the relationship between mental disorder and the sociocultural environment, and aimed to establish the prevalence of all types of mental disturbances whether diagnosed and treated or not; to establish 'who' was mentally disturbed; and to study the aetiology of mental disturbance.

For its time, the survey was sophisticated in its method, giving attention to the representativeness of its sample, and avoiding depending on unreliable existing diagnostic nosology by developing a general impairment scale. From a random sample of 1,911 individuals from the 110,000 residents aged 20–59 in Midtown, 87 per cent (1,600) were successfully interviewed. The study reported a high prevalence of disorder – 23 per cent of the population were judged to be substantially impaired by psychiatric symptoms.

These early epidemiological surveys provided a considerable body of information and drew attention to the importance of psychological and social factors in the aetiology of mental disorder. But they also had limitations. By treating psychiatric disorder as a unified concept rather than as several different disorders, they could not generate rates for different diagnostic groups. Impairment rates were reported independently of diagnosis and therefore obscured diagnostic variations, resulting in a complete lack of information right up to the

1970s on which to base scientific and policy decisions, on the rates of treated and untreated specific psychiatric disorders (Weissman and Klerman, 1978).

With the development of sophisticated standardised assessment procedures, a greater consensus among some of the diverse findings from early epidemiological enquiries became apparent and estimates of the rates for specific disorders became possible. Boyd and Weissman (1981), for instance, re-examined the findings of a large number of early studies and integrated them into the new classifications. They arrived at a lifetime prevalence or overall risk of bipolar affective disorder of between .24 and .88 per 100 for both men and women. The heterogeneous group of non-bipolar depressions, if subsumed into one category of 'a major depressive episode' was considerably more common and affected 3 per cent of men and between 4 per cent and 9 per cent of women at any one time (point prevalence). Recent surveys have found even higher rates, particularly in inner cities. Brown and Harris (1978), using a shortened version of the PSE to calculate the one-year prevalence of depression among women, found it to be 8 per cent in the Outer Hebrides and 15 per cent in Camberwell, South London. About half were new cases (which had begun within the previous twelve months), and about half chronic in the sense of lasting for one year or more. In the same working-class inner-city area of London, Bebbington et al. (1981) reported similarly high rates of disorder on the PSE. Their one-month prevalence was 15 per cent for women, 6 per cent for men. Disorders in both studies were mostly anxiety and depression.

Surtees and his colleagues (1983) also concluded that the point prevalence of psychiatric disorder in women lies between 10 per cent and 15 per cent. In their recent general population survey in Edinburgh they found that depression accounted for the largest proportion of cases (6–9 per cent) and anxiety for most of the rest (2.8–4.5 per cent). However, despite the advances made in assessment techniques, a comparison by these workers of two commonly used methods (CATEGO and RDC) showed quite a wide disagreement between them (Dean et al., 1983). Although they produced prevalence rates of depression and anxiety which were not too discrepant, an examination of the extent to which they picked out the same individuals as cases or non-cases *and* assigned similar diagnoses to those identified was poor. Some of these different diagnoses must be due to the different approaches of the two systems, the RDC taking account of a longer personal history, while the CATEGO imposes time constraints upon the information considered.

What is apparent from all community surveys is that the most prevalent psychiatric disorder is depression, and that many other disorders, particularly among those which do not present to specialist treatment services, have a predominant depressive component.

These studies are all of adults, usually in the age range 20–65 years. Reliable data on older people are more difficult to obtain. Cooper and Sosna (1980) report that both psychiatric case registers and general practice figures give an under-representation of morbidity due to the large numbers of mentally ill old people who live in old folks' homes and nursing homes. Preliminary results of their field study indicate a point prevalence rate of 27 per cent. Organic psychosyndromes (with cognitive disorders) were found in 12 per cent of the sample, mostly aged over 75, while functional mental disorders (affective and neurotic symptoms) were found in 15 per cent. This age group makes little demand on psychiatric services until or unless admission to hospital or other institution becomes unavoidable. Cooper and Sosna found none of their cases were receiving psychiatric treatment and only two cases reported previous episodes of treatment. The majority (78 per cent) had seen their GP within the previous three months, but only 10 per cent were seen by social workers or community nurses.

Compared with the aged, children are a much more easily located age group for community studies. The most extensive and well-known community surveys of psychiatric disorder among children in Britain are those conducted by Rutter and his colleagues on the Isle of Wight and in South London (Rutter et al., 1975a; 1975b). Teachers completed questionnaires on all the children aged between 10 and 11 on a given date with homes on the island or attending schools in one South London borough. Intensive interviews with mothers at home were carried out for selected subgroups. A major discovery was the twofold difference in rates of disorder between London and the Isle of Wight. This difference was examined further in a subsequent paper and is described below. Prevalence rates for psychiatric disorder were found to be 12 per cent in the Isle of Wight and 25.4 per cent in London. Psychiatric disorder in children is defined and assessed in a different way to adult disorder. Most children rated as 'cases' have emotional or behavioural problems.

Community surveys: distribution of illness

The epidemiologist also has the opportunity to obtain a wide range of information on the social and environmental circumstances of each person interviewed. It then becomes possible to look for differences between those people with any given disorder and those without, from which some clues may be derived as to the cause of the disorder. These can provide the starting point for detailed aetiological enquiries. Very often, however, only crude factors on the marital status, age, gender, education and occupation of subjects are collected. Obviously a good deal more detailed information is needed before such information becomes valuable to those seeking prospects for prevention. People cannot avoid being female, old, or widowed for instance. An understanding of what it is about being female that makes women more likely than men to experience psychiatric disorder is needed before this finding becomes of much use.

Demographic variations in the rate of psychiatric disorder which are most commonly reported include a higher rate among women, low social classes, separated and bereaved persons and the unemployed. Bebbington and his colleagues (1981), for instance, interviewed a random sample of 800 Camberwell residents (London), aged 18–64 years. The rate of disorder as assessed by the PSE was more than twice as high among women as men (15 per cent versus 6 per cent). Work outside the home was associated with psychiatric status for both sexes: more than twice as many 'cases' were found among those without jobs. Marital status and the presence of young children in the home was also related to the presence of psychiatric symptoms, but often the association reversed direction for men and women. Married women were found to have over four times as high a rate of psychiatric disorder as single women, and women with children under 15 years at home to have twice the rate of those without. Married men, on the other hand, had less than half the rate of disorder of single men (3 per cent versus 8 per cent), and the rate of disorder among men with children at home was very low. However, for both men and women the demise of a marital relationship (through separation or death) was associated with a high rate of disorder.

Bebbington and his colleagues at first found no relationship between psychiatric disorder and social class for women, although in a later report of the same study (Bebbington *et al.*, 1984) they conclude that there is some evidence that working-class women with young children at home are particularly prone to develop minor psychiatric disorder. This brings them into line with the conclusions of many other community studies which have repeatedly found a higher rate of disturbance among lower social class groups (Dohrenwend and Dohrenwend, 1969). Brown and Harris (1978) established that this was so whether they used their own, the Registrar General's or the Goldthorpe-Hope (Goldthorpe and Hope, 1974) method of determining social class. Twenty-three per cent of working-class women, compared to only 6 per cent of middle-class women among their sample of 458 women in South London, were considered cases in the three months before interview. However, among women who had only recently become depressed, class differences held only for those with children living at home, although chronic cases were more prevalent among working-class women at all life stages and with or without children.

Surtees and his colleagues (1983) have also confirmed that the high rate of psychiatric disorder found in community surveys among working-class women is not attributable either to their methods of determining social class or their diagnostic techniques. Social class of the 577 women interviewed in North East Edinburgh was divided into two groups using two methods – OPCS I, II, III non-manual against III manual, IV and V, and Goldthorpe and Hope groups 1–22 versus groups 23–36. They found that using any of their diagnostic techniques (CATEGO, RDC or Bedford College) and either of the methods for determining social class, there was a much higher prevalence of cases among the working class.

Their study also examined the relationship between rates of psychiatric disorder and three other demographic factors: age, marital and employment status. All three variables were found to be related to psychiatric disorder, whichever diagnostic system was applied. The highest prevalence of disorder was amongst those aged 35–54 although the difference was only statistically significant using the ID–CATEGO system. They also confirmed the relationship between marital status and psychiatric disorder found by other workers – single women have a lower rate of psychiatric illness than married women, while divorced, widowed or separated women have the highest rate. For employment, the highest prevalence was found among those women who did not have jobs outside the home. The difference between employed and unemployed women in prevalence rates was twofold using the RDC and ID, and more than fivefold using the Bedford College definition of cases developed and used by Brown and Harris.

As the four factors were found to be highly inter-related (except age and social class), Surtees and his colleagues examined the extent to which each factor affected morbidity separately, and found that each had an independent effect on prevalence rates. Only age showed differential effects: among the oldest group, the tendency for higher rates among low social classes was reversed; instead, middle-class women had higher rates of disorder. If each variable had an independent effect, it followed that women characterised by a number of these variables would have a particularly high morbidity. This was found to be so, and prevalence ranged from 3.3 per cent (ID) or 6.7 per cent (RDC) for women who were single or married and living with husband, employed and middle-class, to as high as 40 per cent (ID) or 50 per cent (RDC) for women who were widowed, divorced or separated, unemployed and working-class.

Most of the psychiatric disorder identified in these community surveys is characterised by depression and anxiety. The relationships reported between demographic variables and disorder are therefore largely reflecting an association with depressive/anxiety states. And in fact the social correlates of some of the less common disorders are quite different. Murphy (1983) provides a valuable summary. For example, he lists three prominent demographic features of schizophrenia: firstly, that it has a low incidence before the late teens, with onset being later in women than in men; secondly, there is a high percentage of unmarried persons; and thirdly that the prevalence of schizophrenia shows an inverse relationship to social class and status. Rates of the affective psychoses (involving a predominant mood rather than thought disorder) are frequently above average in widows, refugees, military conscripts, inadequately prepared immigrants, mothers whose children have left home, and residents of districts where social interaction is weak, but low in religious communities, and during social movements such as the student protests of the late 1960s.

Of other functional psychoses, Murphy reports that paranoid states arise most commonly in immigrants with little educational knowledge and ability to speak the language; paranoia is more common among males and people of higher educational levels; infantile autism is also more common in higher social or at least educational groups; and the incidence of puerperal psychosis is lower in stable marriages than other family settings, being particularly high among unmarried mothers. The organic psychoses, typified by the senile and the arteriosclerotic group, are more common in developed than developing countries and show some association with social isolation. Persons who move residence in old age are at greater risk, and if the move takes place after onset of the disorder, those people tend to die sooner. Alcoholism is more common among men than women, while women are more likely to become dependent on barbiturates, and more recently on the benzodiazepines (Jones *et al.*, 1984). Amphetamines and cocaine tend to be used most by young people, particularly students (Murphy, 1983).

Many physical and psychosomatic illnesses also show an association with psychosocial variables. And as Murphy notes, it is frequently found that

> mental and somatic illnesses, particularly cardiovascular, tend to
> cluster in the same individuals and that the gravity of any
> somatic illness tends to increase when a mental disturbance,
> particularly depression, is also present. Moreover, even where
> a socio-cultural variation in the distribution of an illness has a
> clearly physical basis, there is often a psychosocial factor
> affecting exposure to that physical element, as for instance in
> lung cancer, where tobacco smoke is the key organic factor but
> where the use of tobacco by some individuals and not others is
> psychosocial.

Demographic factors and treatment

It is often assumed that effective prevention will save money in terms of treatment costs that will be avoided. But it is now well established that most people with psychiatric disorder are never seen by a psychiatrist (Hoeper *et al.*, 1984; Goldberg and Huxley, 1980; Shepherd et al., 1966). This means that it is quite possible that a programme could be quite effective in preventing depression or anxiety, for instance, but have very little effect on the numbers of patients seen by the specialist services. Some indication of the service implications of preventive strategies can be gained from an examination of factors associated with receipt of treatment. Knowledge of the behaviour of people with developing symptoms of disorder is also potentially valuable in that it may reveal opportunities for practitioners to pick up disorders at an earlier stage. Information on the differences between treated and untreated mentally ill people on a range of psychosocial characteristics is easily obtained from epidemiological surveys.

For most people in Britain, their first action when they consider themselves to be ill is to consult their general practitioner. However, a small proportion of mentally ill people will not consult their doctor, and not all of those who do will be recognised as such by the doctor. If a psychiatric diagnosis is given, the GP will then decide whether to treat the patient himself or to refer the patient for psychiatric treatment. The psychiatrist must in his turn decide whether to treat the person as an out-patient or in-patient. Goldberg and Huxley (1980) estimate that while as many as 25 per cent of the general population may be regarded as suffering from some form of psychiatric disturbance in any year, as few as six cases per 1,000 population are represented as in-patient hospital statistics.

Many factors affect a person's likelihood of receiving some form of treatment, including the patient's own confidence in managing his symptoms and his attitude to doctors and psychiatrists, the availability of services, and the attitudes of his relatives. However, the key position of influence is occuped by the GP. To begin with, the GP must recognise the presence of a psychiatric problem. But some people with mental illness describe their problem only in terms of somatic symptoms (such as lack of appetite or problems in sleeping). They may not volunteer information on their psychological symptoms unless the doctor asks a direct question about mental health (Goldberg and Huxley, 1980). This is probably the most common reason why a proportion of psychiatric disorders, particularly mild disorders, are not identified by the general practitioner. Goldberg and Blackwell (1970) asked all patients waiting to see one GP (Blackwell) to complete general health questionnaires. When they compared GHQ scores with the diagnosis of the doctor, they found that for every two psychiatric cases recognised by the physician, a third remained undetected despite having similarly high GHQ scores. Such cases were termed the 'hidden psychiatric morbidity' of general practice.

In addition to their descriptions of their symptoms, certain patient-characteristics make the GP more likely to ascertain a mental illness. Hoeper and his colleagues (1984) compared the ratings of patients on the GHQ to the family doctors' assessment of the patient and found that among those with no previous diagnosis of mental illness, more than twice as many cases were identified by the GHQ as by the doctor (24 per cent against 9 per cent). However, the family doctor was *more* likely than the GHQ to assess a patient as currently having a psychiatric disorder if the patient had a prior history of disorder. Seventy per cent of patients with a previous diagnosis of mental illness were thought by the general practitioner to have a current disorder, while only a third were so rated by the GHQ. This suggests that doctors were mistakenly identifying some patients as mentally ill, particularly as the GHQ is much more accurate in determining the absence of illness than its presence. However, in numerical terms, those with a previous psychiatric history are in the minority, so the more common error is for psychiatric disorder to go unrecognised.

Some of the same factors influence the GP in deciding whether or not to refer a patient he has diagnosed as mentally ill for specialist treatment. Sometimes, however, the effects of patient characteristics have a complex effect on their pathway to care. For instance, women are more likely than men to have their disorders recognised by the GP, but the doctor is less likely to refer a woman than a man to a psychiatrist (Goldberg and Huxley, 1980). Goldberg and Huxley (1980) have reviewed much of the research relating to factors which augment or restrict the individual's passage through the 'filters' on the pathway to in-patient psychiatric treatment (see Table 2.1).

Characteristics of the doctor also affect his accuracy in recognition of disorder: the way in which he interviews his patients, his person-ality, and his academic ability. Ten aspects of the doctor's behaviour in interviewing patients have been found to relate to accuracy, and all can apparently be improved by training. They are: eye contact at outset of interview; clarification of presenting complaint; use of direc-tive questions for physical complaints; starting of interview with open questions and reserving of closed questions for the end of a sequence of questions; empathic style; sensitivity to verbal cues; sensitivity to non-verbal cues; not reading notes during history taking; ability to deal with over-talkativeness; and limitation of questioning about past history (Goldberg and Huxley, 1980).

Given the amount of psychiatric disorder to be seen in general practice, any increased accuracy in identifying disorder could poten-tially place a crippling burden on current services, particularly if many more patients were referred for specialist help. Johnstone and Goldberg (1976) have compared the outcome of disorders left unde-tected and untreated with those brought to the doctor's attention.

Table 2.1 Summary of variables relating to characteristics of the patient determining passage through first three filters

	pass less easily	*pass more easily*
first filter: decision to consult	trivial disorders	severe disorders, many symptoms
	married women with children	stressful life events
	married men	lonely people
	old and poor (USA)	divorced and separated women
		unmarried people
		unemployed
second filter: recognition by the doctor	physical presenting symptoms	severe disorders
	men	women
	below 25; over 65	middle-aged people
	unmarried people	separated, divorced, widowed people
	better educated, students (UK)	seen frequently before
third filter: referred to psychiatrists	mild illness	severe disorders; psychoses
	new, acute and transient women (UK)	more chronic illnesses
		young people
		separated, divorced, widowed women
		unmarried people
		men (UK)
		better educated

(from Goldberg and Huxley, 1980 p. 160).

They used the GHQ as an indicator of probable disorder to identify people with psychiatric symptoms which the general practitioner failed to detect. They found that if the GHQ results were shown to the doctor so that some form of treatment was then offered, the patient tended to make a more rapid recovery than if the doctor remained unaware of the GHQ symptoms. However, even if symptoms remained undetected and untreated, most recovered within twelve months provided they had initially only had a small number of symptoms. But among patients with more than twenty symptoms, those whose general practitioner had seen their GHQ rating continued to fare better one year later. This suggests that a process of screening for psychiatric disorder in general practice, and acting upon that information, may help to reduce prevalence rates. Furthermore, although 'detected' patients increased their consultation for emotional complaints over the ensuing year, they did so at the expense of consultation for physical symptoms, so that their overall consultation rate was not increased (Goldberg and Huxley, 1980).

Demographic studies and aetiology

Many of the studies of the distribution of psychiatric disorder have been carried out by researchers interested in what their correlations might mean in terms of aetiology. They hope to discover what lies behind their statistics. Although research and theory on the origins of depression and schizophrenia are examined in some detail in following chapters, it may be helpful to form a bridge to that research by briefly describing one or two studies which are essentially demographic in nature but which also deal with possible implications for causal processes.

The early study in Midtown Manhattan has already been discussed. The researchers gathered extensive information on the social circumstances of their sample and the analysis showed socioeconomic origin, present socioeconomic status, and age to be highly correlated with mental health ratings, independently of all other factors and of each other (Langner and Michael, 1963). There were also clear differences between treated and untreated cases, the former being wealthier, with more positive attitudes to doctors, better educated and probably with very different diagnostic composition. They also assessed a number of 'stress' factors, including parents' poor mental health, childhood economic deprivation, childhood poor physical health, childhood broken home, parents' character negatively perceived, parental quarrelling, adult poor physical health, poor interpersonal affiliation, work worries and socioeconomic worries. They found that it was less important to mental health risk *which* factors applied than how many. There was an essentially linear relationship between the number of 'stresses' and mental health risk. These stress factors, however, did not account for social class differences in mental health, a finding the authors were unable to explain. That is, the association between low socioeconomic status and poor mental health was independent of the number of stresses experienced. Since this early survey, studies on the role of stress in the aetiology of adult psychiatric disorder have increased dramatically in number.

Researchers like Michael Rutter and his colleagues who demonstrated such marked variations in the rate of childhood psychiatric disorder between London and the Isle of Wight have also speculated about the aetiological significance of 'inner-city stress'. They began by examining the factors within the two populations that were associated with disorder and then went on to look at whether the two regions varied in these same factors (Rutter et al., 1975b).

Four types of variable were found to be associated with disorder: family discord and disruption, parental illness and criminality, and social disadvantage. Those children in severely discordant (unhappy, disruptive, quarrelsome) homes had a higher rate of disorder. Many more children with a psychiatric disorder than 'normal' children had spent at least one week in the care of the local authority (16–19 per cent against 2 per cent). Fathers' anti-social behaviour was associated with disorder in their children: 7 per cent of fathers of disordered children on the Isle of Wight had been in prison at some time, compared to 1 per cent of fathers of normal children (in London the comparison was 20 per cent against 7 per cent). Mothers of disordered children more often had neurotic or depressive disorders than mothers of 'normal' children. Children in large families were more likely than children in smaller families to have psychiatric problems. In both areas, child psychiatric disorder was also more common where fathers had labouring or semi-skilled manual work. Finally, a large number of school variables were found to be correlated with disorder. Where schools were *high* on teacher turnover, pupil turnover, percentage of free meals, absenteeism, percentage of non-indigenous children, and *low* on pupil/staff ratio, they were *higher* in the percentage of deviant children.

The researchers then turned their attention to random sample comparison groups from the two areas. The London sample was found to be considerably worse than the island group in terms of quality of marriage, children in care, mothers' psychiatric disorder, fathers who had been in prison, family size, overcrowding and owning their own home. Similar differences emerged with respect to mothers with psychiatric disorders and school variables. In other words, the prevalence of these variables, shown to be associated with psychiatric disorder in children, largely explained, in a statistical sense at least, the differences found in rates of childhood disorder in London and the Isle of Wight. Large families, discordant marriages, high staff and pupil turnover in schools and so on are all more common in London than in the Isle of Wight, and it is these factors that explain the higher prevalence of disorder in children. The question Rutter and his colleagues were unable to answer, however, is why London mothers should be more depressed, or more commonly experience marital discord.

Sainsbury has made a number of demographic studies of suicide and has speculated about possible economic and social causes. Suicide is linked with psychiatric illness to the extent that it most commonly occurs among people with a history of serious depressive illness or chronic alcoholism (Sainsbury, 1968). Sainsbury makes it clear, however, that people who commit suicide, and those who attempt to do so but live, are on the whole very different populations, although there is some overlap between them. People who unsuccessfully attempt suicide are more likely to suffer from neurotic or personality disorders.

Using data obtained from coroners, Sainsbury found a consistently higher rate of suicide among men than women, both in Britain and many other countries, men with manic depression being at greatest risk. In Britain suicide rates peak in women in their mid-fifties and in men in their mid-sixties. Sainsbury suggests these fluctuations might be associated with people's changing roles at these times. He also found that throughout twenty countries and among all age groups the rate of suicide was higher in the period 1921–2 (a time of relative prosperity) than in the period 1931–3 (a time of world economic depression). Furthermore, the suicide rate changed most among people of high socioeconomic standing, that is, the group who were less likely to lose their livelihood, which led Sainsbury to suggest that the psychological effects of unemployment may have greater causal importance than its financial effects. Another of Sainsbury's findings was that the war years showed a decrease in suicide rates, and he argues in favour of a theory first put forward by Durkheim a century ago that social integration in a community has an important effect on suicide rates.

However, all such claims are at best tentative and many demographic-type studies have assessed psychological and social variables in far too crude a fashion to reveal a great deal about aetiology. Early studies rarely specified the type of psychiatric disorder identified, and without a great deal more data it has only been possible to surmise what it may be about being working-class or female, for instance, that increases the risk for particular diagnoses. There have been many other shortcomings in community psychiatric surveys. Robins (1978) points out that there has been a tendency to avoid questions about promiscuity, violence, drinking and drug problems, and arrest in the mistaken belief that they would not only have been upsetting, but also not answered honestly. According to Robins, such omissions were usual in early epidemiological studies, and by not revealing anti-social behaviour, alcoholism or drug abuse, led to apparently erroneous findings that 'psychiatric disorder' was more common in women than men. Other criticisms of past research made by Robins are of sampling methods – household surveys omit those who die young, those in institutions, and the homeless; of interview methods, which still cannot adequately assess organic brain disease, thought disorder or mental retardation, and are not yet suitably developed for children; the tendency to ignore rare disorders; and of our lack of tools to assess environments.

Weissman and Klerman (1978) also suggest that epidemiological studies should attempt to collect information on biological and genetic factors, hormonal, prenatal and nutritional, for example, as well as on psychosocial factors like life stress, personality and child-hood experiences. Researchers should then establish the relationship (if any) between these 'independent' variables, and the 'dependent' variable, namely, a specific psychiatric disorder. In line with recent developments in genetic transmission and sociology, they encourage an approach which is based on the belief that there is no single causal factor to be discovered, but a number of factors which summate or interact in some way to make the appearance of a clinical disorder highly probable.

A more discriminating approach to epidemiological enquiry would not only help researchers to formulate theories of causation, but would also provide population rates of specific psychiatric disorders. This in turn would improve our ability to evaluate treatment programmes and preventive interventions aimed at specific conditions, to study the use of health services and substantially inform our health planning (Weissman and Klerman, 1978). Of course, although specificity of psychiatric assessment is important if know-ledge is to advance, at the same time it must be acknowledged that current definitions of mental illness rely on operational distinctions and may prove to be inappropriate or in need of further subdivision when understanding of the origins of different disorders advances. Progress will to some extent depend on the validity of definitions and measurement practices now in use. However, research instruments and methods in psychiatric epidemiology have become much more sophisticated in recent years, and this field is at an exciting stage of development. And there appears to have been an encouraging advance in knowledge about aetiology and course of certain disorders.

Conclusions

Research on the social distribution of psychiatric disorders is continuing to throw up a host of interesting associations and valuable aetiological leads. However, cross-sectional studies relying heavily on demographic-type measures which show a positive correlation between social factors and psychiatric disorder can only give us pointers about what might be going on. It is not possible to conclude that because a high percentage of depressed people have a low income, for instance, that lack of money is the cause of the depression and therefore providing more money to low-income families would reduce the incidence of depression. Many other quite different interpretations are equally plausible. The causal sequence may even have been the reverse. A depressed person may have become less prudent in his or her handling of financial matters or less able to obtain well-paid employment. Or a third factor may be responsible for both the poor financial resources and the depression – lack of education, for example, marrying an unsupportive husband, or a particular personality type.

The association simply gives researchers the first clue on the trail to a possible solution. It enables them to develop theories about the nature of the association which can then be tested in more refined enquiries. For the most part, discovering the correlation alone will not provide us with convincing principles on which to found preventive work.

Even if family income *was* found to have a direct effect on psychiatric risk, the expenditure on family income supplements would be unlikely to be measurable in terms of a reduced need for psychiatric services, and perhaps not fully in terms of primary care services either. People over 65 years with psychiatric problems, for instance, are less likely than other age groups to consult their GP, and less likely to be diagnosed as having a psychiatric disorder if they do

(Goldberg and Huxley, 1980; see Table 2.1). Perhaps the GP too often puts down problems of the elderly to their age. The presence of disorder and the effectiveness of preventive programmes therefore needs to be assessed by surveys based on samples drawn randomly from the community.

To test the causal role of a social factor, a time element is needed in the research. It must be possible to find out if the social factor was present *before* the psychiatric disorder. Retrospective studies can add further pieces of the puzzle, but there are inevitably some difficulties in collecting valid information about events which happened a considerable time previously, especially if the person being interviewed is currently mentally ill. Recollections may be coloured by his or her present emotional state.

Prospective research is the ideal way of examining whether a given social factor, present today, causes, or adds to the probability of any particular psychiatric disorder developing at a future date. A sample of people are interviewed at time 1, and re-interviewed at intervals. The development of disorder between time 1 and time 2 can then be studied in relation not only to circumstances prevailing at the time, but also in relation to circumstances at time 1 and which therefore *predated* the emergence of psychiatric problems. However, if disorder is not an immediate consequence, the time lapse may make the exercise both extremely expensive and difficult to carry out. Finally if, as will almost certainly be the case, the disorder is not an inevitable consequence, but follows more often than would be expected by chance, then the circumstances under which it develops need to be pursued. The possible explanations include a biological predisposition of the individual, the particular significance of the social factor in the individual's current circumstances, and/or the chain of events or circumstances brought about by the social factor which increase the likelihood of disorder. These are the complex problems tackled by researchers attempting to explain the causes of mental illness and are described in subsequent chapters.

3
A model for prevention

There are many difficult conceptual issues which need to be clarified at an early stage in reviewing literature relating to prevention. In particular, the whole question of prevention itself can be approached from two quite different perspectives – from that of a disease model or that of a health model.

A disease model

A 'disease modelling' approach to prevention starts from a study of illness and works back to a time when the individual was healthy in the hope of identifying some causal factor which may be open to manipulation. It aims to build up a model of the range of factors which either independently, or more likely by some kind of complex interplay, increase the probability that a person will experience a particular disorder.

The most widely applicable disease model is one of multiple causal factors interacting to produce a particular psychiatric outcome, where

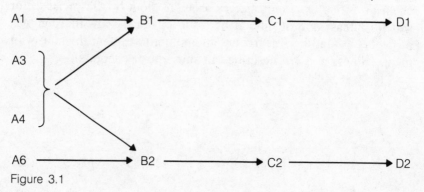

Figure 3.1

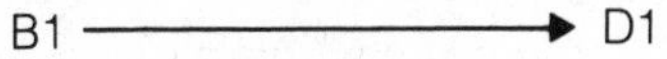

B1 ──────────────→ D1

Figure 3.2

each individual causal factor also has a number of other possible outcomes in other combinations of circumstances.

Figure 3.1, for instance, shows a hypothetical causal chain for two unrelated disorders, D1 and D2. It assumes that there are final common pathways with physiological mediators (C1 and C2). At present these are likely to be poorly understood. There are two kinds of causal factor: one (B) occurs immediately prior to each disorder; and the other (A) is antecedent and linked to the disorder via B. A number of antecedent factors, say A1, A3 and A4, may together in an 'additive' way raise the risk of disorder D1. However, some of these same factors may combine with others to produce the second disorder, D2 (e.g. A3 and A4 may combine with a new factor A6). A third possibility is that one of the factors, say A3, does not increase risk on its own but only in conjunction with some other factor, say A5. On its own A3 has no effect. This, in fact, appears to be an important possibility in the development of psychiatric disorder and will be discussed in terms of *vulnerability*. That is, a vulnerability factor is one that shows little or no effect on its own but increases risk in the presence of another factor.

The simple model of single pathogen B1 leading to disease D1 is rare in physical medicine and even more so in psychiatry (Figure 3.2). Even the common infectious diseases seem usually to be brought about by organisms which are ubiquitous in the environment, which can exist in the body without necessarily producing symptoms, and are most likely to develop into illness when 'host' resistance is impaired. A person's resistance to illness is lower when specific immunity is absent, but may be further impaired by poor general physical health and sometimes even by the effects of social stress. This seems to be true even for a throat infection. For instance Meyer and Haggerty (1962) studied the presence of streptococci in throat cultures from children from fifteen American families over a twelve-month period. Throat cultures were taken every two or three weeks and the acquisition of any new streptococcus noted. Only half of the acquisitions were associated with clinical symptoms of illness. Mothers had been asked to keep a diary of events which disturbed family life over the same period. Distressing events were four times more common just *before* illness or before acquisition without illness than in the two weeks *after* acquisition with or without illness.

The development of most psychiatric disorder is unlikely to be less complex. Furthermore, recent evidence points strongly to the conclusion that it is the meaningfulness of experience that is often critical in the aetiology of a number of psychiatric disorders. This adds yet further complexity, as a stressor no longer can be likened to a microbiological disease agent, although it may still play a comparable role in triggering onset in the aetiological process (Cassel, 1976).

The importance of the use of a disease model and a multifactorial approach for prevention is that they promise to specify fairly accurately those particularly at risk. If, for instance, D1 is equated with clinical depression and A1 with recent bereavement, the risk group – all those recently bereaved – would be large. However, once A3 is identified (say, unexpectedness of the loss) and A4 (say, lack of a supportive network) the size of the risk group will be greatly reduced. The approach is also potentially valuable insofar as it reveals critical points for intervention. In the present example, little can probably be done about the bereavement itself and its degree of expectedness, but the supportiveness of the network may well be subject to influence. To take another example: an important antecedent factor in schizophrenia is an inherited predisposition, yet twins with identical genotypes do not always both develop the illness. (The concordance rate is probably between 40 per cent and 50 per cent (Gottesman and Shields, 1982).) Other antecedent factors must also be at work and these may be more open to intervention.

However, as the method attempts to identify those people at particularly high risk for specific disorders, enabling highly specific preventive approaches for a relatively small population, this also means that the group identified may well already have a number of psychiatric symptoms. For this reason, it is essential that a high threshold for definition of 'caseness' is used. If the threshold is low, then only people who could be described as exceptionally mentally healthy would form the target group for prevention. However, people with minor symptoms often get a great deal worse and in this sense could potentially benefit from preventive intervention. This is not just an academic point. The disease model could be used to identify a high-risk group on the basis of, say, single-parent status and number of children. Many of the high-risk group may well have minor psychiatric symptoms because of the adverse circumstances of their lives. If a threshold for caseness was set so low as to exclude them, because they were deemed already to have a mental illness, then potentially valuable preventive work would be ruled out. This would clearly be absurd. However, this issue has led to some controversy as to whether action to help such high-risk groups is definable as prevention. Throughout this review it will be assumed that a high threshold for definition of 'caseness' is appropriate and therefore that action to alleviate the problems of persons with minor symptomatology can be described as prevention.

Preventive strategies based on such disease models can therefore be formulated by emphasising different points in a causal sequence. In some circumstances it might appear most effective to attempt to eliminate early damaging antecedent factors. Alternatively, attention may be focused on antecedent factors which ameliorate B, so-called 'protective' factors. A third possibility would be to attempt intervention after the risk factors have come together in an effort to interrupt the final process (C) through which they bring about psychiatric illness. This is perhaps best seen in attempts at some general fortifying of the resistance of the 'host'. All have shown some success in the non-psychiatric area, in the many infectious diseases which are now preventable. We have chlorinated water supplies to kill typhus bacteria, and generally improved hygiene standards and food storage requirements to destroy fertile breeding grounds for harmful bacteria, and we have developed immunisation and vaccination so that contact between host and agent does not result in the invasion of the host or the multiplication of the agent (measles, polio, diphtheria, tetanus). The disease model, or one should rather say a number of disease models, have been adopted as the dominant public health paradigm for which they have proved to be admirably suited.

In these examples, however, the preventive methods are aimed at the one essential causal factor to the development of the disorder. They are effectively treating the illnesses as if they conformed to the single agent-single outcome model (Figure 3.2). Undoubtedly this model provides the clearest focus for preventive efforts. There are some psychiatric disorders which approximate to the single-agent/single outcome model, but although preventive opportunities can be identified, there are major difficulties involved in taking the decision to implement them. For instance, Huntington's chorea, which typically begins between age 30 and 50 and progresses inevitably towards dementia, is inherited through a single dominant gene from either parent. But because of the late onset of the disorder and the 50–50 chance of inheritance, a person may not discover his parent has the disorder until he in turn has produced a family. He will not know whether he has the disorder too, and has possibly transmitted it on to his own children, until he reaches middle age. Until now, preventive possibilities have lain only in advising all direct descendants of affected persons against childbearing. However, a genetic marker has recently been discovered which offers the possibility of prediction for relatives at risk of developing the disease (Gusella *et al.*, 1983). This means that those predicted as free of the Huntington's gene would be able to have children with no fear of transmitting the disorder. It might also enable those with the gene to have children free of the disorder if the gene could be detected in the foetus by amniocentesis and pregnancies with an affected foetus terminated. However, the use of such a predictive test would almost certainly create serious psychological problems for those predicted to have the gene. They may well develop a major depressive reaction, and many will undoubtedly decline to be tested (Lloyd, 1985).

There are many other psychiatric disorders in which a genetic factor is present but its most common role is likely to be as a vulnerability factor. Much less is known about the responsible gene or genes and as yet the only preventive possibilities involve counselling people with the disorder, or with a close relative with the disorder, of the probability that their children will develop the condition. However, given the choices involved for the people concerned, it is perhaps not surprising that this method is not as effective as some might think it should be. A prospective study of couples who were at high risk of having a child with a serious disability, such as Down's syndrome, for instance, found that despite counselling advice, a third of the couples were undeterred and planned further pregnancies (Emery *et al.*, 1973).

Of course, in the area of organic-based psychiatric disorder, there have been some impressive results. Half the inmates of Bedlam a century ago would have been suffering from tertiary syphilis. With the prevention and early treatment of sexually transmitted diseases (with penicillin), the prevalence of mental illness from this cause has been dramatically reduced. The dementia of pellagra has been largely prevented by reducing vitamin deficiency with niacin, and lithium has proved valuable in preventing recurrent episodes of mania.

However, most of the psychiatric disorders prevalent today have multifactorial causes, and prevention will need to take account of the complexity of the aetiological process. Investigators using this kind of multifactorial approach are providing potentially valuable information for prevention. Workers based in the MRC Social Psychiatry Research Unit (such as Wing, Brown, Leff, and Vaughn) in London have over a number of years developed an effective biopsychosocial model of schizophrenia which has some similarities to the approach of Strauss and Carpenter (1981) in the United States. Brown and Harris (1978) at Bedford College, London, have developed a psychosocial multifactorial model of depression to which Akiskal (1979) adds a biological dimension. One hope arising from the use of this 'modelling' procedure is that it will reveal at least one factor to enable a ready identification of a 'high-risk' group, and still other factors which may be modifiable in such a way as to reduce risk.

One constellation of antecedent factors which commonly features in studies of psychiatric disorder in the community is stressful events, low social support, low self-esteem and ineffective coping. Given that each may in certain circumstances be modifiable, it is not surprising that a good deal of intervention research has focused on at least some of these elements. But according to the disease model, if action is to have a preventive effect, highly specific information is required about the nature of social support or coping, and the ways in which they may provide protection, the kinds of stress which they may moderate, and the circumstances under which they may be effective. But this is not to say that a full understanding of the entire aetiological process is an essential prerequisite to setting up a preventive programme. The history of prevention in physical medicine reveals a number of instances of the introduction of successful preventive measures (which were *specific* to the disease process) long before the aetiology of the disorder was fully understood. Although these examples are now well known it is perhaps still worth noting that, for instance, more than a hundred years separated the discovery that lime juice prevented scurvy and the identification of vitamin C deficiency; that an East London practitioner was able to reduce the incidence of cholera long before the cholera bacillus was discovered, by removing the handle of a nearby water pump. It is also likely that many clinicians will, through insights gained from long experience, have developed ways of working with psychiatric patients and their families to reduce some of the sources of their vulnerability in their living circumstances and hence reduce their likelihood of relapse.

Their action may be similar to, but have predated, suggestions arising from current aetiological theory. A number of successful preventive methods have undoubtedly been developed from the observations of astute physicians, and they are in an ideal position to carry out some preliminary test of their ideas.

A health perspective

An alternative approach to prevention is to focus instead on helping well people remain as free as possible of symptoms of *any* kind of illness. The underlying rationale derives from the recognition of the ubiquity of ill-health. In effect the findings of research into the causes of specific diseases are restated at a higher level of abstraction. The starting point is that a surprisingly large proportion of the population remain well for much of the time despite the presence of many of the antecedent factors for specific illnesses. Given the range of risk factors, the surprising thing is that anyone remains healthy, not that most people quite often become sick. It is then an easy step to suggest, like Antonovsky (1979), the presence of some overriding factor that is protective for a whole range of possible diseases or disorders.

Advocates of the health approach aim their efforts towards the population as a whole in the context of their everyday lives. The same antecedent factors of Figure 3.1 are of interest, but given the range of ill-health which the factors are capable of producing, details of aetiological processes are of subsidiary interest. People who remain free of significant symptoms are contrasted with those with varying degrees of ill-health. The approach is a positive one in the sense of emphasising resources which facilitate health and growth as opposed to a disease model which searches for noxious agents which might be eliminated or buffered by protective factors.

Health promotion methods include communication, education, legislation, fiscal measures, organisational change, and community development (World Health Organisation, 1984). Common aims are to reduce inequalities in health and access to health care, to develop environments conducive to health and to strengthen community and individual resources to help maintain health.

Although it has its own theoretical approach to research, in practice, surprisingly few original insights and little good quality research have materialised from a health perspective. Most of the information on risk factors which has been taken up by health proponents has been generated by the disease approach – the current campaigns, for instance, against tobacco smoking, high-fat high-sugar diets, and for exercise and a high intake of fibre. An assumption in the health model is that if a factor is less common amongst healthy people, then it is likely to be damaging to everyone, as Bloom (1982) has argued:

> Four vulnerable persons can face a stressful life experience, perhaps the collapse of their marriages, or the loss of their jobs. One person may become severely depressed; the second may subsequently be involved in an automobile accident; the third may become clinically alcoholic; and the fourth may develop a psychotic thought disorder or coronary artery disease.
>
> On the basis of this paradigm, preventive intervention programmes can be organised around facilitating the mastery or reducing the incidence of particular stressful life events without undue regard for the prior specification of which forms of disability might thereby be prevented; that is, this new paradigm begins by abandoning at the outset the search for a unique cause for each disorder.

This quotation illustrates the tendency to generalise about potentially damaging factors, that is, to assume that their effects will almost inevitably lead to one disorder or another. Bloom does not give a fifth, and most common example of a person who remains healthy despite stressful life experiences. Nor does he consider it important to know why the first person experiencing a distressing event might develop depression and the fourth heart disease. He includes the concept of vulnerability in his example, yet is it clear that the assumption is again that the same kind of vulnerability is implicated in a wide range of disorders. Certain factors more commonly found among healthy people are presumed to counterbalance damaging influences. Examples which recur are knowledge, economic security, coping skills and support. Health proponents therefore argue for the reduction of damaging influences, usually environmental and social (e.g. noise, pollution, poor housing, work stress, powerlessness) and the promotion of protective factors (e.g. individual resources).

Of course, whether seeking why people stay healthy from studying the healthy or searching for the aetiological factors of particular disorders, some of the same answers should be discovered. There are several examples where this seems to be happening. For instance, helplessness has been identified as one possible antecedent factor in depression (see chapter 4). People who plan their lives, cope with crises in a masterful way and have a sense of control over the circumstances of their lives seem less likely to develop depression. Antonovksy (1979), an ardent proponent of the study of health (which he suggests should be called 'salutogenesis'), identifies in his fascinating book a similar, though not identical, concept to explain how people remain healthy. He suggests that people have their own personal orientation about the extent to which environments are predictable, and about the likelihood that events will turn out well. This orientation is pervasive, but dynamic, and Antonovsky calls it 'a sense of coherence'. While some disease models have identified helplessness, or in its opposite action, control and mastery, Antonovsky emphasises predictability. Both suggest that a critical variable in remaining healthy is a particular approach to life.

But in disease modelling, it is crucial to specify what it is about any given experience or personal characteristic that links it to any given outcome, that is, to chart the quality and meaning of experience in the context of a person's life. In this way it may become clear, for instance, that if major events are divided into types A and B, and social support into types C and D, that only events of types A and support of type C are implicated in disorder 1, whereas type B events and type D support are, along with a range of other factors, contributing to disorder 2. Disease models would enable identification of a specific risk group and a method of intervention specific to the disorder to which the group were seen to be vulnerable.

Advocates of the health approach would be more interested in predicting risk of ill-health for a population as a whole and mounting programmes on a broad front. There is one puzzling consequence of this strategy. Generalisations about the effects of particular risk factors in this more general fashion will not necessarily be contradicted by evidence marshalled to support rival claims. If, for instance, events of type A and B are put together, and disorder 1 and 2, it is still possible for correlations to emerge even though A events are of no importance for disorder 2 and B events for disorder 1. If correlations are studied at a general level, then major events are linked to a range of disorders. Even social support of a particular kind may prove to be protective to a broad range of disorders although more specific enquiry may show it works in terms of quite different mechanisms. It may, for instance, help to reduce the number of events of aetiological significance to one disorder, and in another have a direct impact on the disorder itself. As soon as correlations are made at a higher, more general level of measurement, then the health-predi- cting approach may produce credible results. Broad correlation studies give rise to the kind of statement made by John Cassel in a much-cited and admired lecture on social support (Cassel, 1976). He pointed to the inappropriateness of the disease model for much psychiatric disorder because most causes are neither sufficient, necessary nor specific. That is, there is little evidence of any factor which will always cause a given psychiatric disorder to develop, or that can be found to be present in the clinical history of every patient, or that will cause one disorder to develop but have no effect on the likelihood of other illnesses developing. He also pointed to the absence of any dose-response relationship, seen in many physical disorders, in which the severity of the risk factor increases likelihood of disease. These statements may well be correct if measurement of risk factors is made at a relatively crude level. Specificity is only revealed when measurement is refined (see chapter 4).

However, disease modelling and health predicting need not be conflicting approaches. Both are necessary: the former to uncover causal factors and test their importance in limited interventions, and the latter to promote those factors which have some general relevance to a wide population. The health model is likely to be particularly relevant in formulating strategies which may alleviate conditions that are very common among the general population. For mild depression and anxiety, for instance, one of the most useful approaches may well be to push for more nursery school places for children of disadvantaged women, for a higher child allowance, better housing, and a reduction in the level of unemployment. And of course it makes sense to try to prevent heart disease through public education campaigns about the dangers of smoking, obesity, high-fat diets and a sedentary life. However, health predicting is unlikely to help in reducing rare conditions such as schizophrenia, where in fact the disease modelling approach has recently begun to pay off by revealing what appear to be highly specific vulnerabilities. And it cannot be ruled out that somewhat surprising vulnerabilities may turn up for some of the more common conditions.

But to return to a point made earlier, disease modelling and health predicting should not be seen as conflicting approaches. Both have their advantages. While disease models provide the most useful information on causal process and risk, medicine is often slow to put such knowledge to use in preventive programmes even after investigators have amassed convincing replications and a number of plausible alternative explanations have been fairly convincingly ruled out. One conclusion of this review is that prevention requires the two sides to come closer, for accurate and practical implications for mental health from disease research to be drawn out and implemented in thoughtful, well-planned and evaluated experimental programmes, a process on which both sides have a poor record.

Focus of this book

I have argued that before generalisable preventive strategies can be formulated and promoted, there must be a fair indication from aetiological research that they could reasonably be expected to be helpful. To answer questions about aetiology and about the possibility of modifying key processes, a disease approach is essential. The overview of evidence on these issues in subsequent chapters therefore focuses on the prevention of illness. Depression and schizophrenia will be used as illustrative examples. Prevention in this context is defined as actions intended to reduce the incidence of mental illness amongst people who are relatively free of distressing psychiatric symptoms or who are suffering from symptoms not extensive and severe enough to be defined as cases. They may never before have experienced mental illness or they may have largely recovered from previous illnesses. This coincides more closely with the lay under-standing of the term, and makes the complex and relatively arbitrary distinctions between primary, secondary and tertiary prevention unnecessary. It also places most treatment issues and methods of reducing the social handicap of chronically mentally ill people firmly outside the scope of this book.

Of course, even with this limited definition of prevention, the literature which can be considered relevant is extensive. Aetiological research, research on social support, crisis management, coping skills, childhood disadvantage, family relationships, stress and many other issues are all relevant. Many years could easily be devoted to the examination of every one of these subjects. The attempt in this book to bring some of the research on these areas together cannot hope to do justice to each of them. Instead, key pieces of research have been selected from each field – studies which seem particularly

important and potentially influential. The aim is to progress by illustration: to fill in the picture in some detail for a few conditions in
the belief that this either has some direct implications for other
conditions or, if not, provides an indication of what might be possible.

There are advantages for a review of this nature in focusing on
definite illness. Any preventive strategies that are revealed are likely
also to have significance for the health of the general population,
and not only those at high risk of mental illness. The reverse is
certainly not true. Many factors that are damaging to the welfare of
the general population will not have causal significance in the genesis
of definite illness. For instance, particular qualities of supportive
relationships have been found to be protective against the effects of
stress and thereby linked to a reduced risk of depression. Other
qualities of relationships seem to be protective against relapse for
those who have suffered from schizophrenia. The same qualities of
support are likely to be conducive to health among the general
population even if their lives are comparatively unstressful and they
have no history of schizophrenia. On the other hand, a host of
distressing circumstances will lead to a wide range of transient mood
disturbances, minor physical ailments and unhappiness which in
most instances would not develop into mental illness. To examine
everything which might be damaging to health would be, at least at
present, an impossible task.

A wide range of psychological, environmental and developmental
factors are implicated in disorders like depression and schizophrenia.
And in most of the literature relating to prevention there seems to
be an implicit assumption that if biological factors are crucial, prevention, on current knowledge at least, is by and large impractical. The
best that could be hoped for is, say, that genetic counselling would
result in a diminution in the numbers of births to women with a high
risk of transmitting disorder to their children. Once an individual
has suffered one major episode of disorder, however, maintenance
drug treatments can be instituted to help reduce the likelihood of
recurrences.

Much of the research and the practical initiatives to prevent
disorder currently focus on the assumption that social factors have a
major causal influence. Yet as recently as 1979, Lamb and Zusman
asserted that there was still a lack of good evidence of a causal
relationship between societal factors and the development of mental
illness. The first task to be undertaken in the review of preventive

literature in the following chapters will therefore be to establish that a reasonable case has already been made for the causal significance of social factors, both in first and recurrent episodes of mental illness.

However, establishing a causal role for any given social factor is not enough. In order to prevent disorder, it must be possible to show that the social circumstances associated with this factor can be modified sufficiently to have an impact on the causal process. This has proved to be far from straightforward. It is easy to think of a whole range of traumatic events that might well precipitate or provoke a psychiatric disorder that could neither have been foreseen nor averted. Furthermore, as discussed in earlier paragraphs, efforts to interrupt the causal sequence require a good deal of information: about the circumstances surrounding the event, the presence of other antecedent factors, and the way the factors come together to colour the interpretation and significance of the event in the context of the person's life. Without such knowledge intervention may well not have the intended effect. The second aim of this review will therefore be to examine the degree to which preventive methods have succeeded in modifying key social factors.

There then remains a third problem, related to the implications of knowledge for services, both those which have hitherto been devoted to the treatment and rehabilitation of people with mental illness, and those concerned with the social welfare and health of the general population. Promising preventive strategies are likely to span many separate professional disciplines and to have implications for community networks, voluntary action and self-help. But without one professional group with primary responsibility for developing preventive mental health approaches, practice may continue as before, whereby help tends to reach only those people with advanced stages of disturbance. This issue will be discussed in the final chapter.

What information is needed in order to prevent psychiatric disorder?

For a consideration of prevention of illness, information is needed about *who* gets ill, *why* they get ill, *when* the process starts and when they might best be helped, *how many* people are affected by particular causal factors, and *how* they may be helped. Differences between people who are 'ill' and those who are not in terms of social, demographic or biological data was reviewed in chapter 2.

To discover whether the risk factors identified really do contribute to the development of disorder or whether there is some other explanation for the association of a particular social factor with mental illness, intensive studies employing sensitive measurements of psychosocial processes are needed. Research must move beyond crude indicators such as whether people are working or unemployed or have large families to examine in detail the context and meaning of such social variables. Very often, things are not as straightforward as they seem.

Take, for instance, the correlational findings on paid employment and women's mental health. There is now a considerable body of evidence to support the contention that paid employment has a beneficial effect compared to being 'only' a housewife (Brown and Harris, 1978; Kessler and McRae, 1981; Bebbington *et al.*, 1981). However, there is other evidence that suggests that women with young children who also work outside the home may experience role conflict and role strain from the difficulties of fulfilling multiple demands. (See, for example, Shimmin *et al.*, 1981; Parry, 1986). These ideas suggest that women's health deteriorates as role strains increase. The level of strain could probably vary according to the number of dependent children, their age, the demands of the employment and the help and support of a partner in sharing parenting and household chores. Finally, there is also the possibility that women with poor health withdraw from the labour market, which could also explain an apparent correlation between good health and paid employment. In fact, Arber and her colleagues (1985) find support for each of these possibilities – that employment can be either protective or damaging depending on the circumstances of the woman, and that chronic ill-health limits labour force participation. It is important, therefore, that causal models are developed which illustrate possible underlying mechanisms. Models and theories on the origins of illness are pursued in chapters 4 and 5.

But even when there is some certainty that a particular social factor does indeed have a causal role in psychiatric disorder, there is often no obvious way of intervening to reduce psychiatric risk. Harris and her colleagues have demonstrated a causal link between a lack of care in childhood, premarital pregnancy, and depression (Harris *et al.*, 1987a; Brown *et al.*, 1986b). But it is unlikely that increasing pregnancy advisory services or even the availability of contraception for girls in such circumstances would do much to reduce the risk of depression. This is because the origins of the vulnerability appear to be at least partly explained by a passive, helpless approach to life. Those girls who unintentionally become pregnant are often those with helpless attitudes who fail to control the difficulties that confront them or to plan their lives in a positive way (Harris *et al.*, 1987b; Rutter, 1982). They are often candidates for depression anyway, although if their circumstances become worsened by falling into an unsatisfactory relationship with the child's father, or finding themselves coping as single parents, the likelihood of depression will be further increased. In such circumstances an improved knowledge of contraception techniques on its own may fail to have much impact.

Many workers in prevention assume that most of the 'causes of the causes' can be traced back to childhood and that primary prevention programmes should therefore be geared towards children. Chapter 6 looks at the evidence for opportunities for effective preventive actions during childhood. But it is equally clear that many health problems among adults often follow distressing events in the person's current life, and occur most frequently among people with chronically stressful living circumstances. For this reason a whole range of services and projects have been developed, often by voluntary groups, to try to help people to cope with the stress they face. Chapter 7 examines the research and theory on life crises, social support and coping. This information is relevant for questions concerning the timing and nature of interventions that are likely to be helpful.

Epidemiological research can give us clues as to why one person seems to be more vulnerable to mental illness than another because of factors in his or her personal life history and current living circumstances. But a different kind of question might be argued to be more relevant to discussions about prevention, and that relates to 'how many?' rather than 'who?'. How many people, for example, are admitted to a particular mental hospital will be strongly influenced by local and national policies. Numbers of available beds will restrict the number of in-patients. But which mentally ill people are placed in those beds will have more to do with the individual circumstances of the patient (how near he is to the hospital, how ill he is, what alternative placements are available). How many people are unemployed is determined by economic policy, regional variations in job opportunities and political decisions. But the answer to the 'who?' question to a certain extent comes down to personal factors: ill-health, old age, poor work skills, low educational attainment (Rutter,

1982). Furthermore, as structural factors become more important, personal factors become less so. When the rate of unemployment is low, personal characteristics which distinguish employed from unemployed persons will be marked. However, as the rate of unemployment increases, the people drawn into the unemployed group will be less and less distinguishable, in terms of personal characteristics, from those with jobs. This is particularly apparent when a major local employer ceases business.

Clearly, structural as well as personal factors must be considered in formulating preventive policies. How many men commit suicide by shooting themselves, or how many teenagers become drug addicts, will be related to the availability and price of guns and drugs. Chapter 8 attempts to broaden the perspective beyond that of the individual and his personal social network to look at the sources of stress in wider societal and cultural practices. It also examines some of the macro-policies which have been implemented aimed at helping those people who are socially at a disadvantage.

Attempts to intervene in people's lives to reduce their likelihood of developing mental illnesses are described in chapter 9. Experimental projects, relevant voluntary initiatives and statutory provision are covered in an attempt to give some overall impression of what is happening in terms of preventive mental health practice at the present time. The evidence which exists on the extent to which preventive goals have been achieved is also discussed. This is perhaps the area where knowledge is most seriously lacking. A final chapter considers some of the problems in translating knowledge into effective practice. While throughout history practice has tended to go far beyond what had reasonably been established in research terms, it is also true that we have not fully implemented the few effective strategies that we know. Furthermore, we have a multitude of as yet unproven but promising leads. The conclusions arrived at in this book concur with those of Rutter (1982) that we need to move ahead to test our hypotheses with trial interventions and evaluate as well as we can what we do.

4
Causes of Depression

Our knowledge of morbid mental states is much less definite
than our knowledge of many physical disturbances. We are not
likely to find a cause as precisely as the tubercle bacillus can be
shown to produce tuberculosis. We find, in every case of mental
disorder, antecedent happenings, no single one of which is the
cause, but all of which contribute. Certainly one is the last
straw, and may be blamed as the exciting factor. But that is often
wrong, because it may be the lightest straw in the whole bundle.
(National Council for Mental Hygiene, 1927)

Depression is the most prevalent of all psychiatric disorders –
described as the common cold of psychiatry. A certain degree of
depression regularly accompanies serious physical illness (Greer,
1985), and one in four working-class women with at least three
young children at home experience clinical depression at some point
during a one-year period (Brown and Harris, 1978). And as
depressed parents can have a deleterious effect on their children's
behaviour and vulnerability to psychiatric disturbance (Rutter, 1966),
the number of people who can be affected in some way by the
disorder is substantial and marks it out as one of the most important
psychiatric conditions. But comparing depression to a cold is
misleading in so much as it implies that the condition is not only
common, but mild. In reality, depression can sometimes be serious
and deadly. Most people who commit suicide are depressed (Robins,
1981), and suicide is one of the top ten causes of death in most
European countries (Kreitman, 1983).

Someone who is mildly depressed finds his everyday life to have
lost its pleasure and interest. Everything requires extra effort and
provides less gratification than before. He feels excessively tired

and preoccupied with ordinary bodily discomforts. Hopes, plans and pleasant memories are hard to keep in mind, and realistic worries take prominence. He can usually continue to work and meet his everyday obligations and may seem normal to acquaintances. But to himself and those close to him, something is not right (Brownsberger *et al.*, 1971).

Someone who is more severely depressed may feel physically ill as well as gloomy. His thinking, speech and movements may be slowed (psychomotor retardation), or he may be tense and restless (agitation). He will quite likely suffer from insomnia, sleeping for short periods, dozing fitfully and perhaps lying awake through the early hours of the morning. These lonely hours may be the time he reaches his deepest despair. He may also lose weight, lose interest in sex and suffer from obscure pains (Brownsberger *et al.*, 1971). The experience has been described as a sense that the self is worthless, the world meaningless and the future pointless (Beck, 1973).

Numerous theories have been formulated to explain the disorder, from many different perspectives: psychoanalytical, social, behavioural, cognitive and biological. Understanding of the disorder has progressed in all these directions, and several attempts have been made to combine some of these ideas in an integrative model (e.g. Akiskal, 1979; Gilbert, 1984). The advantages of the disorder in evolutionary terms have also been considered. Given that natural selection has not eradicated the disorder, despite its association with suicide, with the possibility of reduced fertility, and impaired efficiency in behaviour, it is likely to have had some value. John Price (1968) has made two suggestions: perhaps temporary moods of pessimistic caution have proved to be advantageous in avoiding predators, or perhaps depressive behaviour has evolved as part of the complex behaviour which maintains the stability of man's community. A dominance hierarchy is known to exist in many aggressive animal communities. Perhaps elated behaviour has evolved in connection with a rise in the hierarchy, depressive behaviour with a fall. The causal sequence is unimportant, that is, whether the elation or depression came before or after the rise or fall, as the importance of the behaviour would be that 'he should stay down quietly and not try to make a comeback for some considerable time'!

These ideas may seem fanciful, but Price justifies such speculation as leading us to consider and test new hypotheses which might otherwise not have been considered. For example, the first model would suggest some research into neuroendocrine mechanisms of hibernation in relation to depression; the second to studies of changes in dominance both in animals and man (that is, a person's standing in his group of acquaintances).

In fact, it could be argued that too little has been made of the naturalness of depression – that to a large extent it develops as an understandable reaction to life circumstances. Many theories (conditioning ideas for instance), emphasise the maladaptive aspects of depressive thoughts and behaviour, and the *distortion* by depressed people of the threatfulness of experience. There are likely to be more opportunities for prevention if the social factors themselves *are* of causal significance in clinical depression, rather than the person's distorted interpretation of their threatfulness. And some of the best research evidence on the development of the disorder points towards this conclusion.

Psychoanalytic theories

The similarities and differences between grief and depression have had a central role in the development of psychoanalytic theory. In *Mourning and Melancholia*, published in 1917, Freud proposed that loss was central to both these states. But whereas normal grieving focuses on different aspects of the lost person, the depressed person seems to be grieving over an inner loss. For the depressed person, the loss may be of a more ideal kind and may relate to aspects of himself that destroy his security of self-esteem. He may also be very hostile towards himself, belittling himself. By contrast, self-regard is not usually diminished in normal grieving.

The importance of loss and low self-esteem to depression has been accepted by many. However, there is a good deal of disagreement about how they come about. Freud believed that the depressed person had developed from childhood with high dependency needs. He was therefore always vulnerable to disappointment – since he needed too much, he could never get enough. As Brownsberger and colleagues (1971) describe it

> because his needs are chronically unfulfilled, he has feelings of frustration and anger. Such a person is in a serious bind because expressing his anger will drive away or make hostile the very people he is dependent on. Therefore, he must hold in his

anger, which seems to eat away at his insides, leading ultimately to feelings of helplessness and self-reproach. . . . It usually comes as a surprise to discover how angry the patient is, because superficially and consciously he blames no one but himself.

The cause of the anger is a loss, real or symbolic. The unleashing of the anger against the self causes a catastrophic fall in self-esteem.

Of course, this is a gross oversimplification of a complex and much more wide-ranging theory; a comprehensive review of psychoanalytic ideas can be found elsewhere (see, for example, Ellenberger, 1970; Gilbert, 1984). Only those ideas which can be traced through many different formulations on depression in the seventy years since Freud's book was published are touched upon here.

Many other psychoanalytic theories have been developed since Freud. Some very valuable ideas have been put forward in recent years by John Bowlby (Bowlby, 1969; 1973; 1980). Loss is also central to Bowlby's theory, but the losses which are the basis of vulnerability are real and not imagined and centre on a person's failure to make or maintain a stable and secure relationship with his parents early in childhood. Mourning and depression are not seen as overlapping through different processes; rather, early loss or bereavement actually produces the vulnerability to psychiatric disorder (which may not necessarily be depression). Bowlby's formulations, known as 'attachment theory', suggest a strong causal relationship between the person's early experiences with his parents and his later capacity to make affectionate bonds.

Bowlby believes that we have an instinctive (inherited) need to maintain proximity to attachment figures, because this has had evolutionary survival value. We have therefore developed behaviours designed to maintain proximity to, and protection from, caregivers when those relationships come under threat, such as distress calling and clinging. A range of emotions are consequential upon the making or breaking of close relationships – anger or anxiety when they are threatened, depression when they are lost, joy when they are re-established. Early attachment behaviour is crucial to understanding later psychiatric problems. Certain experiences can predispose a child towards feelings of helplessness, towards a propensity to interpret information in a negative way, and towards a continuing perception of irretrievable loss. For instance, he may have found it impossible to meet his parents' aspirations for him and never attained a secure relationship with them, or he may have repeatedly been told he was unlovable and incompetent, or he may have experienced actual loss of a parent.

Ideas from the psychoanalytical school have been extremely influential, and can be seen to have filtered through into a wide range of theoretical models of depression. In particular, the concepts of loss, attachment, self-esteem, anger against the self and helplessness have been important.

Psychological theories

Both behavioural and cognitive theories are relatively recent developments, and have begun to have some impact only in the last decade or two. Gilbert (1984) provides a valuable summary of many of their approaches. Some of the ideas incorporated in these theories are clearly recognisable from psychoanalytic formulations. But while psychoanalysts often drew many of their ideas from clinical experience with mentally ill patients, many recent psychological approaches have studied how depressive thinking can be induced experimentally in students. This is true of two interesting and important cognitive theories, the first of which has proved to have considerable usefulness in the treatment of depression and the second in understanding some of the biological mediators of depression.

Beck's cognitive theory of depression centres on the development of a negative view of oneself, and life in general, which can lead to depression (Beck, 1973). Once again, childhood loss is seen as the origin of this negative view. The loss may be an object or person, or perhaps an aspiration which held some considerable positive value to the person. If the evaluation of the loss becomes generalised, the person will see himself as a loser, lacking in skills and opportunities to make the future rewarding.

Beck suggests that we have an automatic style of thinking which to a large extent determines the conclusions we derive from experience. The person prone to depression has a tendency to interpret events negatively. However, he does not have this negative interpretation of all events or all the time – otherwise he would be permanently depressed. It is only in the pursuit of important goals that he may see himself in a negative light, and only during the recurrence of situations similar to the childhood loss that brought the negative schema into existence. For instance, the child may have been stigmatised by a physical handicap and rejected by peers for a number of years. In adulthood, he may over-react to rejection from peers – a rebuff from someone he hoped to date perhaps. He would tend to make an extreme and absolute judgment of his worth. He may also learn other negative cognitive schemas. A distressing failure in something which was important to him, athletic ability perhaps, may lead to him making a negative judgment about himself every time he experiences any difficulty in competitive activities in the future. Each time this judgment is made, it reinforces the negative self-image. The key notion is that it is not events themselves which produce depression, but their meaning to the individual person. It is the person's cognitive schema which translates events into their internal representations.

Seligman has also suggested that a maladaptive style of thinking can be learned which predisposes a person to depression. He ident-ifies one particular cognitive style as crucial: helplessness (Seligman, 1975). The theory originates from experiments with rats in which the animals were confined in a small space and given electric shocks. In some instances the rat could learn that, following a particular response, he could prevent the delivery of the electric shock. In others, no response would affect the arrival of the shock. Similar types of set-up were also tried with students confined in a room with a loud noise. The findings were, essentially, that those rats or students receiving the uncontrollable unpleasant experience began by making determined efforts to stop or escape it, but after a lack of success, eventually became passive and helpless. What was of most interest, however, was that these subjects then performed less well in subsequent trials when the outcomes were made controllable than did those animals or students who had previously been in controllable situations.

These findings were considered to have direct implications for the development of depression. 'Learned helplessness' describes the individual's learned expectations that events are largely impervious to his influence and that unpleasant outcomes are probable. This can produce all the negative attributes of depression. These include passivity and intellectual slowness (motivational deficits), a belief that one's actions are doomed to failure (cognitive deficits) and the emotional component of depression. It is not the uncontrollable event, however, which is crucial as a determinant of depression but the *expectation* of a lack of control over stress which is argued to be a sufficient condition for depression (Seligman, 1975).

However, these proposals meant that Beck's and Seligman's explanations were in conflict (Gilbert, 1984). According to Beck's theory people prone to depression have a tendency to blame themselves for negative outcomes. In Seligman's theory, negative outcomes are seen as uncontrollable by the person himself. A good deal of research has been stimulated by the learned helplessness model and by the question of how we attribute causes to different events. Laboratory studies in which researchers have set up tasks in which failure could be induced experimentally have indicated that depressed people have a tendency to blame themselves if they get the task wrong, and the ease of the task if they get it right. This is more in line with Beck's ideas. This and many other weaknesses in Seligman's theory led to a reformulation (Abramson *et al.*, 1978).

The new formulation is based on attribution theory. Attribution theory maintains that the causes of events cannot be observed, but are construed by the individual to render the environment meaningful. The cause may be attributed either to internal factors (self) or external factors (others, the world) and to stable factors (such as ability or task difficulty) or unstable factors (such as luck). Abramson and his colleagues suggest that when a person is unable to resolve a problem he attributes his helplessness to a cause. The cause may be stable or unstable, internal or external, global or specific (that is, extended to all areas of life or felt only in relation to a particular problem). These attributions will determine whether future helplessness will be chronic or acute, broad or narrow, and whether or not self-esteem will be lowered. That is, the generality of the depression will depend on whether the person's helpless views extend to all areas of his life; the length of the depression will depend on how stable his helpless attitudes have become; and self-esteem will be lowered if the person has internalised his helpless attitudes and sees himself as a failure. Finally, they suggest that the intensity of the depression will depend on how strong is the expectation of uncontrollability and on how important the outcome of the situation is seen to be. People who 'typically tend to attribute failure to global, stable and internal factors should be most prone to general and chronic helplessness depression with low self-esteem.' In abandoning the notion that the uncontrollability of events themselves was crucial in favour of personal attributions, the learned helplessness theory is now in line with a cognitive view of depression.

Unusually, Abramson and his colleagues spell out the potential preventive implications of their ideas. First of all, they suggest that it may be possible to identify those people at risk of depression, that is, those who tend to make global, stable and internal attributions for failure, *before* they become depressed. Attempts could then be made to force the person to criticise and change his attributional style. Secondly, people living in social situations likely to produce vulnerability may also be identified, that is, where undesirable outcomes are very probable, and highly desirable outcomes unlikely. Here a change of social circumstances would be needed if vulnerability were to be reduced. Thirdly, it may be possible to help people who have a tendency to exaggerate the unpleasantness or desirability of outcomes not to 'catastrophise' about uncontrollable outcomes. This may reduce the intensity of future depressions. Finally, a life history which encourages people to expect to be able to control the sources of suffering and nurturance in their lives should be protective against depression (Abramson *et al.*, 1978).

This last suggestion has also been made by Garber and her colleagues (1979), who describe several experiments to demonstrate that when people first face controllable unpleasant situations before experiencing uncontrollable unpleasant situations, they are less helpless in later similar circumstances. Thus, if people achieve a fair degree of mastery over outcomes and have experience in controlling and manipulating the sources of reinforcement in their lives before they are exposed to uncontrollability, they should be more resilient to depression. It may be possible to devise some kind of training programme for certain difficulties to achieve this effect.

The model of learned helplessness has many appealing aspects and presents clear avenues for research. Much work has already been generated on the biological mechanisms involved. However, it can by no means be described as a complete model of depression. Furthermore, it has been criticised for not distinguishing between types of depression and confusing sad affect and clinical depression (Buckwald *et al.*, 1978). Most of the work and examples seem far more applicable to the former than to the latter.

Biological components

Adherents to a disease model of mental illness have shown considerable interest in the possibility that disorder is inherited, either a given condition itself, or some related psychological dysfunction. This possibility can best be studied by examining twins growing up together or in different homes. Identical twins have the same genetic constitution and usually a similar upbringing. Fraternal twins have different genetic profiles but a similar upbringing, while identical twins who have not been brought up together will have the same genetic make-up but different social environments. The role of environment and inherited characteristics can then be separately assessed by studying how often both twins with each type of background suffer from psychiatric disorder.

Considerable evidence has accumulated that there is a genetic component to bipolar depressive disorder, that is, where both manic and depressive episodes occur. In 1968, Price reported that the 97 identical and 119 fraternal twin pairs studied up to that date had shown substantially different concordance rates for depression (68 per cent and 23 per cent). Even when environmental factors were controlled by studying identical twins reared apart, the concordance rate remained the same. Severe unipolar depression, that is, depression of a similar type and severity to the bipolar condition, but without alternating swings towards mania, also to some extent seems to run in families. The mode of genetic inheritance is thought to be more complex than for bipolar depression, partly because the morbidity risk for relatives of affected individuals is much lower (Akiskal, 1979). The evidence for genetic inheritance is much less strong for the less severe forms of depression.

There are many ways in which biological factors may be implicated in depression. Erlenmeyer-Kimling (1979) suggests one possible link between genetic and social factors. A good deal of depressive illness is known to follow adverse life events and it is known that human infants show considerable variation in response to separation from their mothers. Suppose a propensity to react more or less negatively to the environment is inherited, but is also affected by environmental circumstances. Two children (A and B) may both inherit a tendency to react negatively to stress. But should A have a childhood characterised by a high degree of stress – a discordant family setting and numerous changes of residence perhaps – he will become increasingly vulnerable to succeeding stresses. If child B has had a relatively unstressful childhood, he will attain adulthood with a lower vulnerability than A. Child C, who also had a stressful upbringing, but inherited a tendency to react much less strongly or negatively to the environment, will also be less vulnerable in adulthood than A. However, there has so far been little cross-fertilisation between research on genetic factors in depression and research on life events.

Knowledge is growing on the physiological effects of life stress. For instance, environmental events can produce alterations in the brain levels of neurotransmitters, particularly serotonin and norepinephrine (see Akiskal, 1979). These transmitters modulate many of the functions impaired by depression – sleep, appetite, motivation, pleasure and so on. A depletion of transmitters is therefore likely to be associated with impaired performance and to render the organism more vulnerable to frustration, loss and other life stresses that are expected to increase adaptive demands. The evidence is complicated and inconclusive, and different types of stress seem to have different effects. Furthermore, the biological factors which predispose certain individuals towards a depletion of these neurotransmitters have not yet been established. However, it may be that for bipolar disorders there is an inherited deficit, while for milder disorders the deficit may come about in other ways (Akiskal, 1979).

Akiskal (1979) has attempted to integrate psychosocial and physiological factors into a unified model of depression. He lists ten factors which he believes research has shown to be related to the incidence of depression: life events; social support; developmental object loss; coping skills; monoamine depletion; monoamine oxidase level; borderline hypothyroid function; impact of puerperium; alcoholism; and familial and genetic factors. He argues that most of these causes are neither necessary nor sufficient, but contributory. He illustrates this point using the life event of separation.

> Separation is not a sufficient cause of depression, because a depressive response of clinical proportions is not observed in more than 10 per cent of those who experience it. . . . Separation is not a necessary cause for depression because many depressions develop in its absence. . . . Separation is not a specific cause for depression, as it precedes the onset or exacerbation of other forms of psychiatric disorder. . . . Separation may result from clinical depression and, therefore,

it may aggravate or maintain a pre-existing depressive condition. . . . Finally, separation may precipitate hospitalisation rather than the depressive disorder.

Each of the factors known to have importance in depression are therefore seen to be contributory and not capable of acting alone in bringing about an episode of depression. All are thought to converge on one 'final common pathway' leading to depression, in the diencephalon of the brain 'as a functional derangement of the neur-ophysiological substrates of reinforcement'. However, as Akiskal has no data to enable him to elaborate on the processes involved or the interaction of the contributing factors, his model does not yet have any practical value.

A psychosocial model of depression

While the psychological and biological theories focus their expla-nations on the person's depressive predisposition, important recent work has been conducted on prevailing environmental factors which bring the psychological factors into play and cause the depression to become manifest. Research on the role of stress in psychiatric disorder has grown markedly since the Second World War when the numbers of psychiatric casualties brought an awareness to the general public of the prevalence of mental illness. As screening procedures prior to recruitment had ensured that mentally ill or emotionally disturbed men were not enlisted, it was reasonable to see stress, rather than predisposition, to be of critical importance (Weissman and Klerman, 1978).

One of the most useful studies of the role of life events and difficulties in depression has been conducted by George Brown and Tirril Harris and their colleagues in London over the last fifteen years. They developed their ideas in part from important work by Paykel and his colleagues on the association between life events and depression and other psychiatric conditions. Paykel was one of the first researchers to categorise life events according to their meaning-fulness and show the qualitative differences between events preceding different disorders (Paykel, 1978). Previously, a quantitive method developed by Holmes and Rahe (1967) was commonly used to describe events, which simply assessed the degree of life change consequent upon them. And much of the theory advanced by Brown and Harris to explain the role of life events in depression drew on the ideas of cognitive psychologists like Beck.

Brown and Harris's model therefore provides a framework within which many of the ideas emanating from different perspectives can be brought together. Biological factors could also easily be incorporated as additional vulnerability factors (see Akiskal, 1979). Furthermore, in emphasising external social factors in the causal process, it provides the most hopeful model for a consideration of prevention, as social factors may be more readily modified than other contributing factors. For these and two other reasons, this model will be described in some detail. Brown and Harris have conducted a series of studies based on intensive interviews with large numbers of women in the community. They are well known for their methodological rigour, and they study factors relating to depression of clinical significance, that is, their cases have symptoms at least as numerous and severe as those treated by psychiatrists in out-patient settings. By contrast, many other formulations lack either systematic research evidence to substantiate them, or their evidence is collected from experimental studies using normal, or perhaps unhappy, students.

Brown and Harris described the foundations of their model and their first major survey in their book *Social Origins of Depression* published in 1978. To begin with, they were largely concerned with the current, rather than past, experiences of their sample of women. They suggested that there are three main sets of aetiological factors in depression: provoking agents, vulnerability factors, and symptom-formation factors. Stressful life events, such as discovering a husband's affair, and long-standing difficulties, such as a husband's continuing unemployment causing financial and marital strains, can often be found to precede the onset of a depressive disorder. Such events and difficulties were termed 'provoking agents'. In order to explain why only some women but not others who experience such problems develop depression, they suggest that other social factors (such as a lack of a confiding relationship in marriage) make some women more vulnerable than others. They suggest that vulnerability factors are usefully conceived as only raising the risk of depression in the presence of a provoking agent. A third set of variables, which will not be discussed here, were included in the model because they influenced the form and severity of the disorder rather than contributing to its onset. These were called 'symptom-formation

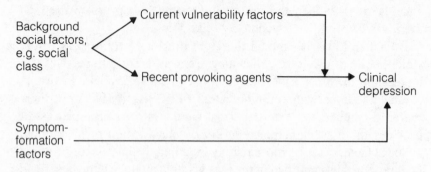

(Source: Brown and Harris, 1978, p. 48)

Figure 4.1

factors'. The model was diagrammatically represented as shown in figure 4.1.

The measure of life events used was one which had been developed by Brown over a number of years and represents a major methodological improvement over previous approaches. It not only enables the categorisation of events in a meaningful way, but also allows the context of the event to be considered. So, for instance, a birth would in all instances have been rated by Holmes and Rahe as entailing a high degree of change. To Paykel, it would have been considered a positive event or 'entrance' event which he would therefore not expect to correlate with depression. But Brown and Harris's Life Event and Difficulties Schedule (LEDS) would not lump all births together in this way. If it was planned and wanted, it would be rated differently to the unplanned birth to an older woman which dashed her plans to take up a job which would enable the family to move to a more satisfactory house.

These ratings of a specific meaning were made possible by a two-stage assessment procedure carried out by the members of the research team, rather than using self-rating questionnaire methods. Interviewers first decided whether a situation was eligible for inclusion by using a set of highly developed criteria provided for them. Secondly, qualities of the event were explored and rated: their characteristics, prior experience and preparation, immediate reactions, consequences and implications. This provided the basis for contextual ratings, the most important of which was found to be long-term threat. Ratings were made by a team of researchers with no knowledge of whether or not the woman was a case, or what she had said about her response to the event. They used their own judgment about how much threat would be involved for most people in those circumstances.

The main part of the study took place in Camberwell, South London. The subjects were women aged eighteen to sixty-five years. One hundred and fourteen residents of the borough who were in-patients or out-patients at three local hospitals, thirty-four depressed women attending local GPs and a random sample (excluding ethnic minorities) of 458 women living in the community were interviewed. All hospital patients had been given a diagnosis of primary depression uncomplicated by any underlying condition such as alcoholism, but were also given a full clinical interview (PSE) by the research psychiatrist. The rest of the women were given a shortened version of the PSE and possible 'cases' were re-interviewed by a psychiatrist. Given that they were not receiving psychiatric treatment, it was important to double-check that their symptoms were indeed similar to those of the women who were. All the women were also given a full social interview about their family, employment, housing, financial circumstances, crises, marital relationship, events and difficulties of the previous twelve months.

The clinical interview provided information about the severity and diagnosis of disorders, but also enabled researchers to measure onset and course using a concept of change-points: a point in time when an increase or decrease in the number of symptoms led to a noticeable change in a woman's psychiatric state. Depressed women were described as onset cases if their symptoms had begun (at a caseness level), at some point during the previous twelve months, and as chronic cases if their symptoms had begun before this. Women with clusters of symptoms not severe or frequent enough to be classified as cases were labelled borderline cases, although some women with one or two symptoms were rated as normal.

The researchers found 17 per cent of their random sample of Camberwell women to be sufficiently severely depressed to be considered cases at some time in the year: 8 per cent onset and 9 per cent chronic. The great majority were suffering from depression. A further 19 per cent of this sample were judged to be borderline cases.

Life events were three times more common among depressed patients and depressed women in the community than among non-depressed women (61 per cent, 68 per cent and 20 per cent), but only if the events constituted a marked or moderate long-term threat and focused on the woman herself or jointly with someone else. These were termed severe events and were assumed to have a causal role. Non-severe events were not more common in patients or onset community cases, and events of extreme severity did not produce depression if their effect was only short-term. Most of the events classified as severe could be interpreted as involving some kind of loss or threat of loss: finding out about a husband's unfaithfulness, a life-threatening illness to someone close, or redundancy from a job held for many years. The loss or disappointment could concern a person or object, a role or an idea. Severe events involving short-term threat, on the other hand, rarely involved loss and were situations where the threat was over within ten days and there were no serious long-term consequences. One example might be where a newborn child developed an infection requiring special care, but recovered in a few days.

The onset of depression usually followed a severe event quite rapidly – within a matter of weeks and sometimes even days. However, there was some evidence that events could act over a period as long as six months or even a year, particularly in the patient series. Furthermore, evidence was described to support their contention that the events were of formative importance, and were not merely serving to trigger depression in a woman who would shortly have become depressed anyway.

Brown and Harris found that it was not only discrete events which could provoke depression. Long-term difficulties were capable of playing a similar role. Problems like overcrowded home conditions or a husband's alcoholism, which had been going on for at least two years and which were rated as major difficulties (1–3 on a 6-point scale of severity), were found to occur in the lives of a great many more psychiatric cases than normal women. Two-thirds of both patients and community cases experienced major difficulties compared to only 20 per cent of the sample of normal women.

However, only one in five of the women who experienced a severe life event or major difficulty subsequently developed depression. The authors therefore examined the data for explanations as to why some women were more vulnerable than others, or, expressed another way, why some women seemed resilient to, or protected from, or were able to cope with adversity such that they did not develop clinical depression.

Four 'vulnerability' factors were identified: the absence of a close, intimate, confiding relationship with someone; loss of mother through separation or death before the age of eleven years; three or more children under fifteen years living at home; the absence of a job outside the home. The model predicts that vulnerability factors can only be expected to be revealed amongst women experiencing major difficulties or who have recently experienced a severe event. The percentages quoted are therefore proportions only of the women who were classed as having a provoking agent.

Among the random sample of women in Camberwell experiencing a severe event or major difficulty, only 10 per cent of those with a close, confiding relationship with their husband or boyfriend developed depression. This compared with 26 per cent of the women without an intimate tie with husband or boyfriend, but who reported a confiding relationship with another person (seen at least weekly), and with 41 per cent of those who had a confidante seen less than weekly or who had no such relationship at all. Loss of mother, through separation or death, was a second vulnerability factor: 47 per cent of women who had lost their mother against 17 per cent of remaining women developed depression following a provoking factor during the year under study. And comparing those women with three or more children at home against those with fewer or no children, 43 per cent and 17 per cent respectively became depressed. Finally, having a job outside the home decreased vulnerability. The effect of this factor, however, could only be detected when the other vulnerability factors were also considered. Among women protected by a close, confiding relationship with their husband, not having a job was unimportant and did not increase their vulnerability. Those who were already more vulnerable, however, due to lack of such a relationship, were half as likely to develop depression following a provoking agent if they worked outside the home. If they also experienced one of the other two vulnerability factors, having a job again afforded some protective effect. All of the women without a confiding relationship or a job who also experienced one of the other vulnerability factors became depressed. Of the four factors, a confiding tie with a husband or lover was seen to be the most important, in that this could protect against depression whether or not any one of the other three vulnerability factors was present.

These vulnerability factors were identified among the random sample of women in Camberwell. A comparison of those women who had become hospital patients with women in the community who were not depressed did not, however, fully replicate these findings. In particular, the depressed patients did not have a substantially higher rate of early loss of mother, nor were they much more likely to have three or more children at home. The authors argue that this is not evidence that their model is incorrect or inapplicable to treated cases, but that, to a certain extent, the factors which make women vulnerable to depression also make them less likely to receive psychiatric help. Among women in the general population, having three or more children at home was found to increase a woman's vulnerability to depression in the face of provoking agents. But it is easy to accept Brown and Harris's cautious suggestion that this same factor may make it difficult for the woman to get treatment. To begin with, a general practitioner may be less likely to diagnose her symptoms as depression, seeing tiredness and other problems as understandable consequences of looking after three young children. He or she, and, for that matter, the woman herself, may also feel it is likely to be difficult for her to be able to attend a hospital out-patient department. If this interpretation is correct, this will mean that women with children will be under-represented among treated patient samples. As a statistical association was found between having three or more children at home and the early loss factor, this might also help to explain the lower rate of early loss among treated patients when compared with cases identified in the community.

When the authors looked at the proportion of the community experiencing vulnerability factors, important social class differences emerged. Working-class women were found to have more vulnerability factors than middle-class women, which largely explained class differences in the rate of depression.

Having established their basic model, the authors go on to describe their speculative theory of the processes involved (see Figure 4.2). Two main concepts are crucial: self-esteem and hopelessness. They suggest that any average person would have some feelings of hopelessness in response to the sorts of provoking agents they describe, but that women with low self-esteem would be less able to handle such feelings and more likely to allow them to generalise. The vulnerability factors are argued to contribute to low self-esteem, or, as protective factors, to high self-esteem. This is why vulnerability factors only become of causal significance when a severe event occurs or major difficulties exist. A close relationship was thought to provide a sense of being valued. Hence the lack of an intimate relationship, or the presence of a critical and uninterested husband, was suggested

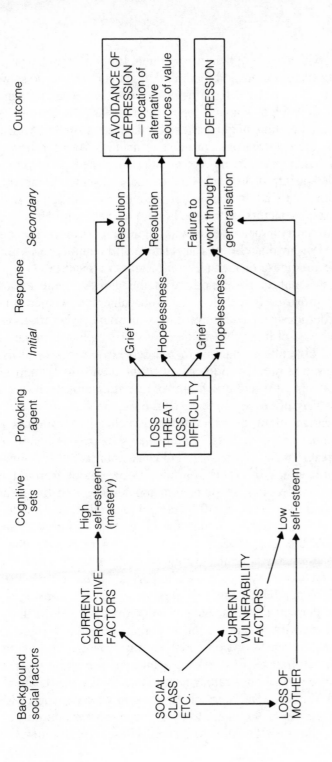

Background
social factors

Cognitive
sets

Provoking
agent

Response

Initial

Secondary

Outcome

CURRENT
PROTECTIVE
FACTORS

High
self-esteem
(mastery)

LOSS
THREAT
LOSS
DIFFICULTY

Grief

Hopelessness

Resolution

Resolution

AVOIDANCE OF
DEPRESSION
— location of
alternative
sources of value

SOCIAL
CLASS
ETC.

CURRENT
VULNERABILITY
FACTORS

Low
self-esteem

Grief

Hopelessness

Failure to
work through

generalisation

DEPRESSION

LOSS OF
MOTHER

(Source: Brown and Harris, 1978)

Figure 4.2   Schematic outline of causal model (capitals) of depression and theoretical interpretations (small type)

as associated with a sense of being less valued. In such circumstances, social activities or a job outside the home might compensate to some extent by providing alternative sources of value. But three or more children would limit a woman's opportunities for social activities considerably. One child might easily be taken along or left with a babysitter. Three children present more difficulties. And not having experienced 'good enough' mothering was suggested as setting a long-term personality of low self-confidence. To some extent, this factor was linked to adult depression through its association with other vulnerability factors. Perhaps the lack of self-confidence led the woman to marry a man she knew to be unsupportive in case she was not asked by anyone else. Perhaps she lacked confidence to find a job outside the house or manage contraception efficiently.

Depression is not an all-or-nothing matter, however, and events which might provoke clinical depression in vulnerable women may produce borderline-case depressive illness in women who are more protected in terms of these four factors. Some examples of the kinds of events and difficulties which provoked depressive illnesses in the sample are given in the Appendix. Many of the events do not appear to be amenable to prevention. Some of the difficulties, however, could clearly very often be reduced, or the woman's ability to cope with them enhanced by being introduced to helping resources – grants for home improvements, arrangements to pay off debts in more manageable ways, or marriage guidance counselling. Furthermore, while the effects of events in producing depression were often so rapid that there would scarcely be time to intervene after the event and before depression, major difficulties, by definition, had existed for at least two years, giving ample time for preventive intervention. In fact many of the severe events arose out of long-term difficulties.

There are also many potential avenues for prevention through the vulnerability factors, and it would seem important to discover whether in practice vulnerability can be modified through preventive programmes. Perhaps during social education discussions in schools, more emphasis could be put on the importance of considering the long-term supportiveness of a potential marriage partner, of thinking through one's aspirations for work and children and taking positive steps to achieve one's hopes rather than letting things 'just happen'. There could be more awareness of the ways in which women with children can get out of the home to meet socially or take up outside employment, and more facilities to increase those opportunities.

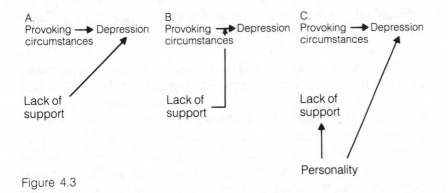

Figure 4.3

A psychoevolutionary perspective

A rival theory concerning the role of close relationships in depression to the Brown and Harris model has been put forward by Scott Henderson. He developed his original perspective from Bowlby's ideas about man's instinctive needs to maintain close attachments. The evolutionary advantage of pair bonding to protect offspring and male group relationships to facilitate hunting is well recognised. Henderson's theory therefore centred on the belief that a lack of social relationships is atypical, that an inability to form social ties is disadvantageous, and the loss of or non-availability of important others likely to be emotionally distressing (Henderson, 1974). Depressive symptoms are interpreted as abnormal 'care-eliciting behaviour' – behaviour intended to bring important others closer when a person perceives himself deficient in the receipt of care. After several cross-sectional studies with colleagues, he carried out a large-scale prospective enquiry in Canberra (Henderson *et al.*, 1980). He expected to demonstrate that social support was related to depression independently of stress (Figure 4.3A).

People lacking supportive relationships were expected to be prone to depression whether or not they experienced major difficulties or threatening events. Alternative models are that support is protective against depression only when people have disturbing events or living circumstances and otherwise is unrelated to depression, as suggested by Brown and Harris (Figure 4.3B). Or it could be related to a third confounding variable such as personality and this latter variable related to risk of depression (Figure 4.3C). An example of 4.3C would be if a person's withdrawn, defensive personality made it difficult for her to establish close friendships, and if those same characteristics of personality, rather than her lack of friendships, made her prone to depression.

Using the General Health Questionnaire and their own measures of social interaction and of recent life experiences, Henderson and his colleagues interviewed a large random sample of adults in Canberra. The measure of social interaction rated the availability of six provisions of social relationships: attachment, social integration, opportunity for nurturing others, reassurance of worth, a sense of reliable alliance and the obtaining of help and guidance. It also enabled an assessment of the adequacy of the provisions in the eyes of the respondent.

A modest negative association was found between neurotic symptoms and availability of attachment and social integration. However, a much stronger negative association was found between neurotic symptoms and the perceived adequacy of social relationships. It also seemed that the perceived adequacy of close relationships was of most importance to women, while for men it was the perceived adequacy of more diffuse relationships that was crucial.

In the longitudinal part of the enquiry, the investigators examined the possible causal role of support. They interviewed a random subsample of 323 adults at four-month intervals on three further occasions. A lack of social support at the first interview was found to be associated with the presence of psychiatric symptoms (GHQ scores) at the second interview among those who had initially been well (GHQ score less than 4). There was a much smaller association between adversity measured at the first interview and symptoms at the second. They therefore concluded that a lack of social relationships was a causal factor in the onset of neurosis. However, the relationship between symptoms and support was stronger when adversity was higher, disproving their expectation that support was important independently of adversity.

Because their correlations were strongly linked to their rating of the respondent's perceived adequacy of their social relationships but not to their availability, they conclude that it is not therefore the actual social environment of people which is important to the development of neurotic symptoms, but rather that, when faced with adversity, it is those individuals who view their social relationships as inadequate who have a substantially increased risk of developing neurotic symptoms. From their results they argue that this is not so much an objective assessment of the functioning of their personal networks, but a judgment based on the 'intrapsychic needs of the respondent, in terms of "dependency" or anxious attachment' (Henderson, 1982).

In other words, it is the personality of the individual which is crucial (as in Figure 4.3C). This line of argument is bound to be disappointing for those looking at aetiological studies in search of implications for prevention. It means that 'attributes of the individual which are biological or constitutional are likely to be more powerful than properties of the immediate social environment or other ecological variables' (Henderson, 1982, p. 228.) It means that the reason there seems to be an association between low social support and vulnerability to neurosis is because the same attributes of personality that make a person vulnerable to depression also make a person see their friends and relatives as unhelpful, whether or not they are around and available to help. So we have the disappointing conclusion, from the point of view of prevention, that people with a neurotic type of personality are more likely than other people to develop clinical neurotic symptoms when faced with adversity. But we are given no clues as to why some people should develop such personality traits. As it stands, the crucial implication of these findings, if they are correct, is that increasing the availability of support for people with adverse living circumstances in an attempt to prevent depression would not be expected to be effective.

These fundamental differences in the explanations of Brown and Harris and those of Henderson and his colleagues about the role of social support in the aetiology of depression have prompted a search for the reasons for their discrepant findings. O'Connor and Brown (1984) suggested that one explanation may be that Henderson did not differentiate between the actual support provided in terms of confiding and frequency of contact and the attachment felt for the person named. They argue that the people to whom one feels most attached will not necessarily be those who provide support. O'Connor and Brown maintain that truly supportive relationships (frequent contact and high level of confiding) reinforce a positive evaluation of self and are protective of mental health. On the other hand, feelings of attachment to a person named as very close are not related to either. In a study by this research team of married women in North London, feelings of attachment were not associated with self-esteem or depressive symptoms. A second point, raised by Brown and his colleagues (1986c) concerned the decision by Henderson to analyse the role of support only for those women completely free from any psychiatric symptoms. This may also have caused the effects of support to be obscured. Many women with adverse living circumstances at the first interview will have had one or two psychiatric symptoms and would be particularly likely to benefit from social support. The existence of these symptoms, however, will have caused these women to be omitted from Henderson's analysis. But perhaps what these discussions about Henderson's research illustrate most graphically is the considerable conceptual and methodological difficulty of conducting research on social support. These issues will be discussed further in chapter 7.

Social and psychological factors relating to vulnerability and onset: evidence

It is clear that Brown and Harris's model of depression provides the most scope for preventive formulations, that it is the most complete model of depression available, and has been most systematically researched. Henderson's alternative explanations have not been substantiated, but Brown and Harris's basic model has been confirmed and supplemented in further studies both in Islington in London and in a rural community in North West Scotland, and the original findings have been replicated by other investigators in other areas (see Brown and Harris, 1986 for a recent review). What other evidence is there to confirm the importance of some of these factors?

(i) Life events

An increased rate of major events has repeatedly been demonstrated to occur in a period prior to the onset or recurrence of a variety of psychiatric disorders (Dohrenwend and Dohrenwend, 1974; Lazarus and Cohen, 1977; Brown and Harris, 1978; Paykel, 1978; Kennedy *et al.*, 1983). Follow-up studies of people experiencing particularly traumatic events such as bereavement have also shown a high rate of associated depression and anxiety. For instance, Parkes and Brown (1972) interviewed sixty-eight young people in Boston on three occasions during the year after they had been bereaved. Compared to a matched sample of non-bereaved people, more of the bereaved received hospital treatment and experienced disturbance of sleep, appetite and weight. Their consumption of tranquillisers, alcohol and tobacco increased and their income fell. Up to fourteen months after the event, bereaved persons still showed more depression and a higher incidence of autonomic symptoms (dizziness, fainting, trembling, nervousness, chest pain, sweating and palpitations).

Paykel (1979) describes his research in New Haven in which the life experiences of 185 depressed patients receiving hospital treatment were compared with the experiences of a random sample of the same number of adults in the general population over a six-month period. He tried various ways of categorising events – as desirable (arrival of a wanted new baby) or undesirable (compulsory redundancy) or according to whether they represented exits from or entrances to the subject's life. Patients reported about three times as many undesirable events in the six months preceding their illness as the comparison group over the same period. There were no group differences for events rated as desirable. If the same events were re-categorised as 'exits' or 'entrances', a similar pattern emerged: exit events were more common among the depressed group, but entrance events showed no group differences. Interpersonal arguments and difficulties were also a more common feature of the experiences of depressed patients than of the comparison group.

Further evidence to suggest that events are important in depression according to their threatfulness rather than according to the amount of change they signify comes from a study by Tennant and Andrews (1978). They interviewed a random sample of eighty-six people in Sydney about recent life events, and used the General Health Questionnaire (GHQ) to gather information about any psychiatric symptoms. They found a closer association between GHQ scores and events when those events were categorised according to their emotionally distressing impact than according to change in lifestyle.

However, these kinds of events are not only of importance in depression; they are implicated in a variety of illnesses. Paykel (1979) pointed out that events are also more common in the lives of schizophrenic patients in the six months before their first admission and in the six months prior to suicide attempts. In fact, in his research, suicide attempters reported the most events, followed by people with depression, then those suffering from schizophrenia, and lastly the general population. The exit-entrance distinction was found to be more specific for depression, and people who attempted suicide not only had an excess of exit events, but also an excess of entrance events. People who had attempted suicide were also particularly likely to have experienced an excess of events beyond their own control, which were rated as undesirable, and scaled as major or intermediate in terms of upset. However, Paykel argues that specificity is, at best, weak, and therefore concludes that the same events may result in a variety of disturbances. Other investigations have made a link between events and onset of physical disturbances such as an infarct, streptococcal infection, and gastrointestinal disorder (see Craig and Brown, 1984).

However, it appears that when the measurement both of the disorder and of the type of event are attempted at a high level of specificity, then more specific correlations are revealed. There is some evidence that particular characteristics of events are more likely to be implicated in one disorder than another. For instance, Finlay-Jones and Brown (1981) were able to show a markedly higher rate of events characterised by danger in the lives of general practice patients suffering from a recent onset of anxiety or from a mixture of anxiety and depression than in the lives of depressed and non-case patients. Events characterised by loss, on the other hand, were more commonly experienced by patients with a depressive disorder.

One of the pitfalls of this kind of research is that, far from events causing a particular disorder, the causal sequence may actually be the reverse. That is, the insidious onset of the disorder and tendency of the person to behave in an unusual way brings about certain events like changes of jobs or relationships before more obvious symptoms of disorder appear. This possibility can be guarded against by distinguishing between independent and dependent events. Independent events are those which are most unlikely to have been brought about by the behaviour of the respondent, such as a husband's car accident which happened while the woman was at home. Finlay-Jones and Brown found the relationship between loss events and depression and between danger events and anxiety remained after dependent and possibly dependent events were removed from the analysis. This encouraged the authors to argue for some causal role for these specific event types.

The magnitude of the link between events and depression has been estimated in various ways. Paykel (1979) calculated that the risk of a person developing depression increases sixfold in the six months following an exit event. Tennant and Andrews (1978) used their Australian sample to calculate that if social support and a person's coping skills were poor, and their stress scores high, then their risk of neurosis was over 40 per cent. But even these figures can be misleading in the same way as would a statistic relating risk of lung cancer as a percentage of all smokers. A very small proportion of cigarette smokers develop lung cancer, but almost all people with lung cancer are or have been smokers. This is similar to the position on life events. Less than one in five people experiencing a severely threatening event or long-term difficulties will develop depression (Brown and Harris, 1978), but from a review of ten community surveys of depression using the same Life Event and Difficulty Schedule, Brown et al. (1987) found at least 76 per cent of depressive illness in the general population to be brought on by severe events or major difficulties.

However, there has been considerable controversy over the meaning of the link between events and depression – whether in fact the existence of a psychosocial stressor makes a depressive response so understandable that it should not be considered a disease. Following this logic, only those depressive conditions where a stressor is apparently absent should be considered as 'real' depression, which is also sometimes assumed to be more likely to include psychotic symptoms and biological dysfunction. This is a long-running debate which will not be documented here. But it now seems to be established that there is no clear-cut difference in the role of environmental factors in so-called 'neurotic' or 'psychotic' depressions (see Paykel et al., 1984). But the important consideration for prevention is the identification of methods of intervention which will make serious depressive illnesses less likely to occur. It is relatively unimportant what these conditions are called as long as they are characterised by a sufficient number of symptoms of depression to be definable as cases. Psychosocial stressors are common enough in such conditions to warrant attention. While a number of depressive illnesses treated by psychiatrists seem to have no link with environmental stress, many more do. Furthermore, Calloway et al. (1984a; 1984b) found that depressed patients with the most clear signs of biological dysfunction had no less chance of having an antecedent stressor.

Paykel (1979) provides a useful model to describe the process by which life events can lead to physical or psychological disorder (see Figure 4.4). Firstly, the significance of the event in terms of its meaning is important. Then other current stresses and supports in the social environment may moderate its consequences, such as

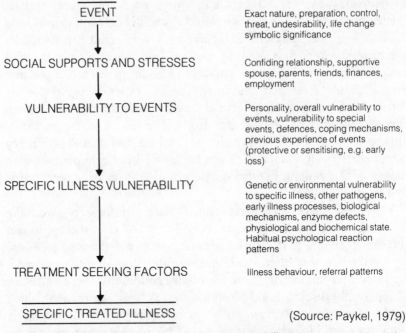

Figure 4.4   Modifying factors between event and illness

outside employment and confiding relationships. Paykel separates
these from the person's specific vulnerability to events, or to
particular events, which has developed from personality attributes
or developmental experiences. Vulnerability to specific illnesses, of
genetic or environmental origin, will also sensitise a person to
particular types of events. Finally, illness behaviour will determine
whether or not the individual regards himself as ill and seeks
professional treatment.

This approach takes into consideration the person's past history
and current circumstances which may cause them to be especially
susceptible to respond adversely to particular types of event. The
person may also have other genetic or environmental reasons to be
susceptible to one type of disorder rather than another. This idea,
that the event is of particular significance when it matches the vulnerability of the individual, has recently been further amplified by Brown
and his colleagues (1987), following a longitudinal study of
depression among women in Islington, North London. They found
that a severe event was of most aetiological significance if it threatened a role, person or idea to which a woman was particularly

committed (established in an interview one year before) or if it matched a long-standing major difficulty in the woman's life. For example, a woman highly committed to her parenting role would be particularly sensitive to an event which threatened her view of herself as a good mother, such as discovering her child had been regularly truanting from school. Had she been less committed to parenting, perhaps because her children were older and seen to be less in need of her support, or had it been an event which threatened a role or idea to which she was less committed, perhaps losing a part-time job which she did not enjoy, the effect would be less threatening. Similarly, events arising out of long-standing difficulties would increase risk of depression: where, for instance, a husband left home after years of arguing and discord; a child was arrested for burglary after a long history of behavioural problems at home and school; or a substantial fine was incurred after a long period of extreme financial difficulty (Brown *et al.*, 1987).

(ii)   Past loss

There is a long history of concern for the potential significance of childhood parental loss through separation or death, and the development of emotional and behavioural problems in childhood and later life. John Bowlby's discussions about the fundamental importance of a continuous, warm mother-child relationship to mental health have been particularly influential over the last three decades (Bowlby, 1951; 1969; 1973; 1980). A large number of empirical studies have attempted to confirm this link. Despite the volume of research, however, the relationship has remained in doubt. Some of the studies have demonstrated a clear association, others show no relationship, while the findings of others have been equivocal. Investigators who have reviewed the research have come to quite opposite conclusions. Granville-Grossman (1968) examined seventeen studies on parental death, ten of which used a control group, and seven studies on parental deprivation (that is, broken homes due to parental death *or* separation). Because, in numerical terms, fewer showed a relationship with depression than those which failed to do so, he concludes that the relationship is probably absent. Some years later, Crook and Elliot (1980) conducted a similar review and came to similar conclusions, suggesting that social class is a confounding variable that has led to a spurious association in some studies between loss and depression.

On the other hand, Birtchnell (1970) and Nelson (1982) disagree. Nelson reviewed sixteen studies on early parental death, severity of depression and attempted suicide and came to the conclusion that a relationship between early loss and severe depression and with attempted suicide *has* been established. The studies examined were all controlled ones with samples divided according to severity of depression and controlling for age, social class and sex. Nelson argues that the failure of other reviewers to come to the same conclusion was because they used vague definitions of depression and failed to take into account the severity of the disorder. Brown and his colleagues (1986a) have also pointed out that many studies have failed to take into account the current circumstances of their samples. If, as Brown and Harris (1978) suggested, early loss acts as a vulnerability factor, rather than being of aetiological significance in its own right, then the relationship between loss and depression would be expected to be strongest in the presence of a psychosocial stressor. Samples with relatively unstressful lives would probably fail to show a higher rate of depression among those with early loss.

A recent study by Brown and his colleagues (1986b) in Walthamstow, North London, was set up specifically to explore the intervening links between childhood parental loss and adult depression. If their earlier positive results could be replicated, then it was important to study how early loss could increase vulnerability to depression. There seemed to be at least two possible mechanisms. The external circumstances surrounding the loss, such as the disruption caused or discordant family relationships leading up to the loss, may be the most important factors, as Rutter (1981) has argued. Bowlby (1980), on the other hand, gave greatest weight to the disruption of the mother-child bond, which he suggested led to particular 'cognitive biases'. These biases, resulting from disordered mourning, might involve compulsive caregiving to others, ambivalence and anxiety in relationships, or a show of independence from close ties. Of course, both external and internal factors of this kind may be operating. The external factors, like an unhappy home setting and difficulties associated with living with one parent, could indirectly raise the risk of depression by making unwise choices more likely – early marriage, or dropping out of school, perhaps – and hence leading to higher levels of adverse life events. The internal factors, leading to cognitive biases, might result in poorer relationships, less self-esteem, and more helplessness. These in turn could again both contribute to vulnerability and increase the occurrence of adverse events.

A sample of 225 women was selected from general practice registers to include a large number of women who had lost a parent in childhood. The interviews covered the psychiatric history of each woman, current psychiatric state, and detailed information about their loss of parent and parenting arrangements which followed. The importance of loss of mother to rates of adult depression was confirmed. Depression in the previous twelve months was experienced by three times more women who had experienced maternal loss or separation (of at least one year) in childhood than by women with no such childhood experiences. Death of father was unrelated to adult depression, although separation from father was associated with a slightly raised risk of depression.

Summarising a complex analysis of a good deal of qualitative data, two factors emerged as of particular importance in linking childhood parental loss and adult depression: the quality of the caring relationship which followed the loss, and teenage relationships with the opposite sex. An examination of the parenting arrangements following loss of mother showed that indifference and a low level of control had characterised the childhood experiences of a number of the women found to be depressed. These two aspects – marked or moderate parental indifference (neglect, lack of interest and attention), and low parental control – were combined into an index of 'lack of care'. Firstly, lack of care was associated with at least a threefold increase in the risk of depression, whether the women were working-class or middle-class, and whether the loss was by separation or by death. Secondly, a much higher proportion of working-class women experiencing early loss and premarital pregnancy (PMP) were found to be depressed than women in the same group without PMP. Among middle-class women, early marriage played a similar role in increasing risk of depression.

Early sexual relationships and lack of care were associated with each other in increasing the risk of depression. For example, early marriage only raised the risk of depression for middle-class women if lack of care had also been experienced, and lack of care, particularly institutional care, raised the risk of premarital pregnancy occurring. One other linking factor then became important with respect to PMP, namely, how the young woman dealt with the situation. Those coping

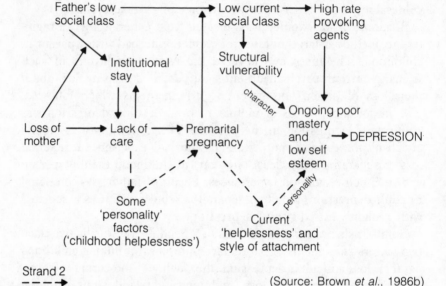

Figure 4.5   Causal model showing main lines of impact of loss of mother

effectively, who decided to marry the child's father for other reasons besides the pregnancy, or who arranged adoption or termination of pregnancy, were less likely to become depressed. Many more middle-class than working-class girls fell into this group, which was thought to explain why PMP seemed less important for them. Those who coped less effectively, and allowed themselves to become trapped into unsatisfactory lifestyles, were found to be more likely to become depressed, perhaps because they had reduced their chances of achieving a dependable, intimate relationship with their husband, or increased their chances of stressful lives. Finally, there also seemed to be some evidence than an internal bias towards helplessness (similar to Seligman's concept) was implicated at some stage, in making PMP more likely or leading to poor coping responses.

From all these complex intervening circumstances, they conclude that two strands of influence will have an impact on self-esteem and the development of depression following childhood loss (Fig. 4.5).

This model shows one route linking early loss to depression for working-class women through premarital pregnancy, and poor coping, making continued working-class status more likely. As such they are ultimately subject to a higher rate of vulnerability factors and provoking agents. In particular, they will often have an unsatisfactory marital relationship, a factor central to a woman's vulnerability to depression.

The second strand shows the link between the cognitive sets and coping styles which develop from 'lack of care' when it occurs following loss of mother. Thus the alternate routes could be seen either as a personality pathway or an experience pathway, which are probably closely interrelated.

A further study by this research team, in Islington, North London, has confirmed that the importance of maternal loss is explained by the quality of care following loss. In fact, a lack of care was found to be a vulnerability factor in the absence of maternal loss, while the reverse was not true. They interviewed nearly 400 women, approximately half of whom had experienced a recent provoking agent. One-third of those with childhood lack of care were depressed, compared to one-sixth of those without lack of care. Considering loss of mother without controlling for lack of care did not produce a statistically significant difference in their rate of depression (Bifulco, *et al.*, 1987). This is a particularly interesting finding from the point of view of prevention as it indicates a much larger risk group. The number of people who as children were separated from their mother, or whose mother died, is likely to be relatively small. Many more children, however, will be subject to a lack of care in the terms described by these researchers.

(iii) Premarital pregnancy and institutional care

The model showing the significance of loss of mother to adult depression by Brown and his colleagues given above suggests that not only is loss of mother an independent vulnerability factor in the aetiology of depression, but that both premarital pregnancy and institutional care could also be considered as vulnerability factors (see Harris *et al.*, 1987a). They are considered together here because of their close association with each other – girls experiencing institutional care also show a particularly high rate of premarital pregnancy (Quinton *et al.*, 1984).

Over the last twelve years, Quinton and Rutter and their research team in London have collected a considerable amount of fascinating information in their study of the links between childhood experiences and parenting behaviour (with special reference to children received into the care of the local authority). This research is of particular importance for a consideration of prevention because the findings demonstrate a clear link between a very similar notion of childhood lack of care to that of Brown and his colleagues, premarital pregnancy and later emotional vulnerability and psychosocial difficulty, but also show that the chain of adverse experience tends to continue into successive generations. Lack of care is often repeated: ex-care women in their study were considerably more likely than a comparison group to suffer a breakdown in their own role as parents, resulting in one in five of their children also being admitted into institutional care. The wealth of qualitative data collected in this research reveals a number of valuable clues for prevention in the life history of children experiencing poor parenting. For this reason it will be described in some detail.

Eighty girls who had lived in one of two children's homes in 1964, when they had been subjects of a study by Jack Tizard and his colleagues, were traced and interviewed by Quinton and his colleagues, when they were aged between twenty-one and twenty-seven years. A similar-aged comparison group of women was found who had also participated in a previous study. Information on childhood history, family, peer and work experiences was obtained, as well as detailed information on current circumstances.

Comparing the two groups of women, twice as many of those reared in an institution had become pregnant and given birth to a surviving child by the follow-up interview. And two-fifths of the ex-care women had become pregnant before the age of nineteen years, while none of the comparison group had done so. Marked differences also existed in their relationships with the father of their children: less than two-thirds of the ex-care women but all the comparison women were living with the father of their child. Serious failures in parenting were also evident in the ex-care sample: one-fifth of their children had been taken into care and as many as one-third of the women had experienced some form of transient or permanent parenting breakdown with at least one of their children. This occurred with none of the comparison group mothers. Parenting breakdown meant that the child had been looked after by someone other than its mother for at least six months.

There were also substantial group differences in parenting at the time of the interview. Parenting was described as 'poor' if there was a marked lack of warmth or a low sensitivity to the child's needs and difficulties in at least two of the three areas of disciplinary control (consistency, effectiveness, style), and as 'good' if none of these difficulties occurred. Two-fifths of the ex-care sample had a rating of poor parenting, compared to one in nine of the comparison group. Observational data confirmed these findings, as do the results of other studies. For example, in their intensive observations of mothers with their first born 20-week old babies, Wolkind et al. (1977) found that those women who had been separated from either or both of their own parents in the context of a disrupted early family life interacted with their babies considerably less than the rest of the mothers.

The ex-care women studied by Quinton and his colleagues were not only more likely to have parenting problems than other women, however. They also had a wide range of other social problems. In particular they had considerably more marital difficulties, and were much more likely to be currently suffering from psychiatric disorder. These findings were similar to the results of an earlier retrospective study by the same research team of forty-eight families who had a child (aged five to eight years) admitted into residential care (Quinton and Rutter, 1984a; 1984b). The mothers of children admitted into care expressed less warmth and showed less sensitivity in their parenting, and their child control was less effective, than in a comparison group of families. They were more likely to be single mothers, have large families and poor housing circumstances (sharing beds, no play space). Both mothers and fathers of children admitted into care were more likely than a comparison group to have a psychiatric disorder. The researchers concluded from these two studies that parenting problems were brought about through long-standing problems in social relationships. Many mothers with parenting difficulties had a long history of emotional problems themselves, and seemed generally lacking in sensitivity to their children's anxieties and needs rather than deficient in specific child management techniques. Taken together, the two studies suggest a causal role for the experience of poor parenting in childhood in later poor psychosocial functioning.

However, a substantial minority (31 per cent) of the ex-care women studied prospectively showed 'good' parenting (Quinton et al., 1984). A number of factors could be identified which helped to explain the apparent resilience of these women. Firstly, positive school experiences were found to be important. They were rated as positive if the subject had two or more of: examination success; a positive assessment of school work or relationships with peers; or a clearly positive recall of at least three aspects of school life. Forty-three per cent of ex-care girls without positive experiences, compared to 6 per cent of those with positive experiences, had poor social functioning in adult life. The relationship also held for parenting. However, positive school experiences were not related to outcome among the comparison sample.

Secondly, the events which followed the girls' departure from institutional care were important. Those returning to a discordant family environment were much more likely to become pregnant than those who returned to a harmonious family or remained in the institution until achieving independence. Ninety-three per cent of the discordant family subgroup had a child (often as a teenager) compared to 51 per cent of those remaining in the institution, and 30 per cent of those going to harmonious families. The adverse circumstances appeared to be part of a chain of events: girls experiencing early disrupted parenting before being admitted into care were most likely to return from the institution to a discordant home. They were then at even higher risk for teenage pregnancy and marrying for a negative reason (i.e. to escape stressful circumstances or because an unwanted marriage was forced by pregnancy). The chain continued, as quality of parenting was also found to be associated with the presence or absence of a supportive marital relationship, and whether or not the spouse also showed psychosocial problems. Unfortunately, ex-care women were much less likely to experience the protective effect of a non-deviant supportive spouse, firstly because they were more likely than comparison women to marry men with problems, and secondly because they were much more likely to be without any kind of spouse.

A harmonious relationship with a non-deviant spouse was more likely among those who planned their marriage or cohabitation. 'Planning' was judged to have taken place if the girl had known the man for at least six months before cohabitation and if she cohabited for positive reasons rather than because of outside pressures such as pregnancy or the need to escape from an unhappy home. Girls who reported positive experiences at school were much more likely to be 'planners'.

The discussion which followed their results is very much in line with the ideas of Brown and Harris. Quinton and his colleagues suggest that girls with positive experiences of school acquire a sense of their own worth and of their ability to control their own destinies, which in turn helps them to cope and resolve their difficulties and plan their own future. The comparison group of girls had many other sources of self-esteem, which was why a positive school experience was much less important to them. Childhood adversities also affect parenting indirectly through their effects on choice of spouse. If, however, through planning or chance, the women ended up with a supportive non-deviant spouse, they were no more likely to experience parenting problems than the comparison group of women. The adverse childhood experiences therefore seemed to act in two ways. They increased the likelihood of a chain of events which put the woman into a position in adult life where she was more likely to experience further social difficulties. They also acted to decrease the woman's coping skills, making her more likely to become depressed or a less sensitive parent when faced with social difficulties or a lack of marital support.

Quinton and his colleagues point out that there are therefore a number of opportunities to break the chain of adverse circumstances, and suggest several potentially fruitful areas for intervention. The first occurs at the transition from the institution to independence, when the girls were often in need of help and about to launch themselves on a course in life from which it might be hard to turn back. Advice and support at this time could aim to minimise the chances of a girl returning to an unhappy discordant home and to parents with whom she may largely have lost touch. This would remove the incentive to marry as an escape from an intolerable environment. A second possibility would be to try to help the individual to become a 'planner'. Institutional rearing and other adverse childhood experience is liable to produce a feeling that one is in the hands of fate, thus anything to increase the young person's social problem-solving skills and their belief in their own ability to control what happens to them might be helpful. Children at school need to be able to find a range of opportunities to derive self-esteem other than from academic achievement, and to have social conditions conducive to establishing good peer group relationships. Sex education needs to be educational in the broadest sense and encourage foresight in all aspects of life, discouraging feelings of hopelessness and inevitability. Thus they emphasise the need 'to focus on personal changes that will enhance self-esteem, self-efficacy and confidence, and increase coping skills . . . and on environmental changes that will increase opportunites and make it more likely that later social circumstances will be beneficial'.

Thus both Quinton and Rutter (1983) and Brown and Harris and their colleagues (Harris *et al.*, 1987a) have shown that pregnancies are more common amongst girls with childhood lack of care than in a comparison group. Both have also documented a high level of family discord in the homes these girls left and to which they sometimes returned. Both have charted important links between these adverse childhood experiences and adult psychosocial functioning. Brown and Harris have illustrated the extent of the link with psychiatric disorder. Of the sixteen women in their survey who were currently working-class and had been in institutional care, ten had premarital pregnancies. Seven of these ten were clinically depressed at interview. Two others (of the sixteen) were also depressed, so out of the nine who had been in care and were currently depressed, seven had also had premarital pregnancies. Premarital pregnancy was therefore almost invariably a link between institutional care and later depression. In Quinton and Rutter's sample, 42 per cent of ex-care girls had already become pregnant by the age of nineteen years.

Both these studies have emphasised the importance to these women of marrying supportive husbands, which markedly increases their chances of avoiding parenting difficulties and depression. Both conclude that a supportive marital relationship (and Quinton and Rutter would add 'past positive experience of schooling') act as a protective factor when a woman is facing marked social difficulties. There are close similarities too in the factors suggested by these investigators as leading to good marriages. Brown and Harris highlight the girl's success in coping with her premarital pregnancy, Quinton and Rutter her planning ability. Both emphasise the role of feelings of helplessness, of behaving as if one is a victim of fate, as important in the process leading to a range of adult psychosocial difficulties. There would seem to be ample justification for preventive interventions aimed at reducing feelings of helplessness, if it were possible, and of enhancing feelings of self-esteem for women raised in institutions or for other reasons experiencing a marked lack of care in childhood.

Both of these important studies describe childhood lack of care as the starting point for a life history of misfortune and a high risk of depression. If the chain is unbroken and poor parenting and depression results, the same sequence of events may well be replicated in the next generation.

5
Origins of schizophrenia

Schizophrenia is primarily a thought disorder, whereas depression is dominated by a mood disorder. It is described as a psychosis, which is characterised by a distortion in the person's perception of reality. In psychotic disorder, thinking, emotions, attention and communication can be affected, seriously interfering with the person's ability to function in a way which might be considered normal. Hallucinations and delusions are common features. Cutting (1985) has collected a number of personal accounts of people's early subjective experiences of the condition. The following illustrates many of the perceptual disorders which may occur:

> There was a tremendous feeling of claustrophobia, of being trapped. Traffic was too loud. Too many people on the pavement. Walls were moving in on me. I'd panic when the house was getting too small, then I'd go outside. But outside the noise was too great. Nowhere, nowhere I could cope. Not even safe in bed ... All the bright colours frightened me most, orange and red ... I recognised people everywhere ... I had all these thoughts in my head but when I spoke it was just noise, just high-pitched noises came out. It had lost its meaning. I could understand other people's language but not my own. (Remitted schizophrenic, in Cutting, 1985, p. 182)

Schizophrenia is also currently defined as a functional psychosis. This description assumes that the disorder cannot be attributed to any known specific abnormality of the brain. As such, schizophrenia can be distinguished from progressive degeneration disorders of the brain like senile dementia, the delirium or dementia which may sometimes follow severe head injury or drug abuse, and the effects of neurological conditions like Huntington's chorea or brain tumours.

Like depression, schizophrenia can take different forms. One person may function well in most areas of life, but be paranoid and hostile in certain circumstances. Another may be bizarre in manner and appearance, passive and withdrawn. Such differences have encouraged the view, which has been held by many psychiatrists since the disorder was first identified, that schizophrenia is in fact a group of related conditions. These conditions are assumed to have the same final common pathway of biochemical interactions, and lead to a similar series of consequences (Warner, 1985).

Unlike the situation for depression, however, only the barest bones of a model have yet been developed to describe its aetiology. Research and theory on the origins of schizophrenia have developed simultaneously in a number of very different directions which can broadly be categorised as genetic, organic and psychosocial. Each decade since the turn of the century has seen influence swing from one camp to the other (see Cutting, 1985). In the 1940s an interest in genetic studies came to the fore, although several German investigators had already been following this line for some years. Geneticists produced and analysed statistics, primarily relating to morbidity levels among relatives of individuals suffering from schizophrenia. Twins were often studied to chart how often both would develop the condition. By contrast, environmentalists often focused instead on the meanings of the symptoms they observed in their patients, and drew attention to the rearing and experiential difficulties a person may have undergone during their formative and developmental years. During the 1950s those seeking organic explanations were encouraged by the discovery of similarities between schizophrenia and the effects of hallucinatory drugs like LSD, and by the efficacy of the newly introduced neuroleptic drugs. A host of aetiological hypotheses has been formed, which have frequently been untestable and based on data that had been unsystematically selected or of dubious validity (Rosenthal, 1968).

The conference in 1968 on the transmission of schizophrenia, reported by Rosenthal and Kety, brought together researchers from each camp, and is probably the time at which all sides came to agree that both genetic and environmental factors must be implicated in some way. It is now generally agreed that some kind of predisposition to schizophrenia is inherited, but that certain environmental factors will increase the likelihood that the disorder will occur and recur. Interestingly, much of the psychological research is now being used to argue for an organic cause. The information about the difficulties of conveying the intended meaning of language, and about the problems in memory and attention experienced by many people with schizophrenia, has been combined with neuropsychological knowledge to suggest the possibility of a dysfunction of one of the two hemispheres of the brain, probably the right side (Cutting, 1985). The evidence for genetic, organic and psychosocial factors in the development of schizophrenia is summarised below.

Genetic evidence

A number of studies have now firmly established the existence of a genetic component in the transmission of schizophrenia. Kestenbaum (1980) quotes the lifetime risk of developing the disorder as between 0.8 per cent and 1 per cent in the general population, which rises to 13 per cent for a child with one schizophrenic parent, and to 35– 40 per cent for a child with two schizophrenic parents. The twin studies conducted by Gottesman and Shields (1972) found a concordance rate among identical twins (that is, the frequency with which both twins develop the disorder) of 42 per cent, compared to 9 per cent for fraternal twins and siblings. Rosenthal's work in Denmark has also been very influential. He has studied the offspring of women with a history of schizophrenia who have been adopted by non-schizophrenic mothers. He found that these adopted children still developed schizophrenia more often than a comparison group of adopted children whose biological mothers had no known record of mental illness (Rosenthal, 1968). This means that the high rate of schizophrenia among close relatives of an affected person cannot be explained away in terms of the effects of living with someone with schizophrenia, and any unusual relationship which might have developed between them. Rosenthal's own research, and his review of other genetic studies, also leads him to argue that the high probability that identical twins will either both develop or both remain free of schizophrenia is explained by their identical genetic constitution, rather than by a tendency on the part of their friends, relatives and parents to behave towards each of them in a very similar way. Rosenthal points out, however, that although these studies have established a genetic component, over half the twins (50–60 per cent) with the same genotype as their schizophrenic partners do *not* develop schizophrenia. It cannot therefore be described as an inherited disease. The feeling is, rather, that a certain genetic vulnerability is inherited which may or may not lead to schizophrenia.

The exact method of genetic transmission is still controversial. Different investigators have argued for a partial dominant gene, a two-gene theory, a polygenic theory, and a combination of genes of incompatible traits. A single gene may be responsible in that although the identical twin concordance rate is only 40–50 per cent, there has been some suggestion that the other twin often has some schizoid features of personality which may be the same disease in a much milder form (Emery, 1975). Other facts, however, such as a much lower than expected rate in more distant relatives, make a single gene theory seem unlikely. On current evidence, polygenic inheritance is the most likely mechanism (Cutting, 1985). Among children at high risk of developing schizophrenia, that is, those with a first-degree relative with the illness, there are as yet no reliable means of predicting whether or not they will also develop the disorder. Research is continuing into possible immunological, biochemical and psychological markers.

Given that the involvement of genetic factors is no longer in dispute, two questions need to be answered. Firstly, just what is it that is inherited, and secondly, how and which environmental factors cause the disorder to become manifest? The answer to both these questions remains unresolved, but a good deal of informed speculation has been generated.

Organic causes

A great deal of research evidence points to some kind of organic disorder in schizophrenia, but its causal significance is unclear. There are essentially three groups of differences between the brains of people with schizophrenia and the brains of non-schizophrenic persons: anatomical, biochemical and functional. There is also a well-established link between schizophrenia and a number of physical conditions, including epilepsy, Huntington's chorea, virus infection, trauma at birth and head injury in adulthood (Cutting, 1985). Firstly, there are anatomical reports of ventricular enlargement and cortical atrophy in people with chronic schizophrenia, and of a thickening of the corpus collosum and cerebral atrophy (Cutting, 1985). The most important evidence relating to such differences has come from CT brain scans (computed tomography), which have shown appearances suggestive of slight cerebral atrophy in at least a quarter of schizo-phrenic patients in varying diagnostic subgroups and at varying stages of the disorder. This particular difference is not, therefore, thought to be confined to one subtype of the illness, or to be a result of treatment procedures (Warner, 1985). It may, however, be an indi-cator of some earlier brain injury (perhaps from obstetric compli-cations or viral infection) which served to increase the vulnerability of the person to schizophrenia. However, it should perhaps be made clear that for most people with schizophrenia, their brains appear completely normal as far as can be made out when looked at under the microscope.

Secondly, biochemical differences in schizophrenia certainly exist, but then they also exist between people who are angry and those who are watching television. But particular abnormalities in biochemistry have been linked to schizophrenia since it was first discovered that hallucinatory drugs could induce a psychosis. The most well-known biochemical theory relates to the activity of one of the neurotransmit-ters, dopamine, at the synapses between nerves. Since emotion and thought are regulated by a complex system of transmissions between nerve cells, and since acute stress can lead to an increase in dopamine turnover, this could in theory precipitate a psychotic episode. However, there is so far only scant evidence to support this hypothesis.

Thirdly, there have been a number of studies which have found abnormal levels of arousal and an inability to maintain attention among people with schizophrenia. Heart rate and skin conductance have been used as measures of arousal, and unusually high levels have been reported (e.g. Venables, 1964). Responses in experimental tests, such as reacting to one of a range of flashing lights, have been used to study selective attention. It seems that people with a history of schizophrenia may also have some difficulty in ignoring irrelevant stimuli (such as other distracting flashing lights), and therefore in maintaining concentration. These two attributes together would mean that a high level of stress would cause the individual to become overwhelmed. The need of schizophrenic patients to sometimes with-draw would then be explicable as a protective response from further stimulation.

The anatomical differences revealed by CT scans have also been found to correspond to the development of schizophrenia in identical twins. Enlarged ventricles have been found in an identical twin who develops schizophrenia, compared to the one who does not. This has encouraged Cutting (1985) to argue that schizophrenia represents an imbalance of the brain hemispheres, that is, that the right hemisphere is dysfunctional and its contribution to mental life diminished, while the left hemisphere becomes relatively more active and dominates the right. Certainly, this hypothesis fits the evidence well. It would explain the abnormalities of emotion and language, because of the specialisation in function of the two hemispheres. The right hemisphere is more concerned with emotion than the left and therefore its dysfunction would explain many characteristic features of emotion disorder in schizophrenia. The left hemisphere is responsible for the construction of spoken language, but the right contributes to its intended meaning. Thus hemisphere imbalance again fits the data well, since the most outstanding disorder of language in schizophrenia is a reduced ability to convey intended meaning, while phonemes and syntax are largely undisturbed. Cutting's thesis of right hemisphere dysfunction and left hemisphere overactivation can also explain the characteristic disorders of attention, perception and thought.

Hemisphere imbalance may seem to explain schizophrenic symptoms, but like a good deal of the information on the development of schizophrenia, it has not yet been backed up by a convincing aetiological model. Cutting has only two suggestions for how hemisphere imbalance might arise, neither of which are pursued in his book. He believes perinatal trauma to be a likely contributing factor, because this in theory could produce damage to the right hemisphere. He also suggests that right hemisphere dysfunction may be inherited, and perinatal brain damage may increase the likelihood of this becoming clinically apparent in later life. He argues that the imbalance acts to increase the person's risk of schizophrenia by making him or her more susceptible to social influences (Cutting, 1985, p. 391). But just how genetic, organic and social factors interact is not at all clear.

Psychological causes

Many psychological theories have grown out of the observations of the often abnormal communication styles of families of schizophrenic patients. The factors argued to have causal significance have included: the family's effect on the child's ability to maintain attention; linguistic disturbances of parents; decision-making processes;

and overprotection. The conference in 1968 reported by Rosenthal and Kety concluded that none of these factors had yet been convincingly established as having a causal role. The situation has not much changed. In 1975 Hirsch and Leff produced a scholarly review of the literature on abnormalities in family interactions. They drew on studies of individual cases, questionnaire surveys, studies of the interactions of parents of people with schizophrenia in small group situations, data from tests of abnormal thought processes of parents, and of abnormalities of their communication and language. From these they summarised what they judged to have been established.

Firstly, they found from eight of the better designed studies that 'mothers of schizophrenics are more concerned, protective, and possibly more intrusive than control mothers both in the current situation and in their attitudes to the children before they showed signs of schizophrenia'. They noted, however, that it was possible that excessive protectiveness could result from having an abnormal child rather than the reverse. Apart from possible personality abnormalities, there is evidence that individuals who later develop schizophrenia more frequently suffered ill-health or mild disability in early childhood than other children. Secondly, they found a large number of studies which showed that parents of people with schizophrenia have greater marital disharmony than controls. Disharmony is indicated by open or tacit conflict, expressed hostility, opposition of spontaneously expressed attitudes, and difficulty in reaching agreement. Thirdly, several of the studies focusing on mothers of people with schizophrenia showed them to be more likely to be psychiatrically disturbed, and in particular, more schizoid than mothers of normal children. Once again, this association might be explained as the consequence of bringing up a child vulnerable to schizophrenia.

Finally, studies investigating the communication styles of parents were found to produce conflicting results. However, one of the more sophisticated studies seemed to indicate that parents of people with schizophrenia *can* be reliably differentiated from the parents neurotics or normals. This work, by Singer and Wynne (1966), demonstrated communication abnormalities characterised by disruptions, vagueness, irrelevance and lack of closure (such as answering with a question or giving contradictory information). These communication styles can be expected to induce difficulties in the listener's ability to focus attention and handle the meaning of what is being said. They describe some typical conversations in which comments from

one person did not link in an expected way to preceding comments
– where there seemed to be a very loose connection between what
one person said and the next. The effects were believed to have
enduring consequences on the child's thought processes and predispose to (rather than precipitate) schizophrenia. However, Hirsch and
Leff's attempt to replicate this study, also reported in their book
(1975), failed to find the same degree of gross communication
disorder as that claimed by Singer and Wynne. They did, however,
find a higher rate of deviance in communication style, particularly
among fathers, which was largely accounted for by overtalkativeness.
Although some bizarre interchanges therefore seem to be real occur-
rences in these families, the research has so far been unable to
convincingly demonstrate a causal link between such communication
abnormalities and the development of schizophrenia in the child.

Prospective studies throw more light on the antecedent factors but
only one study has followed up high-risk young people for a sufficient
number of years to provide any helpful analyses. In 1962 Mednick
and Schulsinger in Copenhagen examined 207 high-risk children,
born between 1941 and 1954, whose mothers had chronic severe
schizophrenia. They also studied a comparison group of 104 subjects
(a low-risk group, children of normal mothers). By 1967, twenty of
the sample had experienced one of a variety of psychiatric disturbances ranging from schizophrenia, to extreme schizoid states, to anti-
social behaviour. Mednick and his colleagues (1981a) describe four
characteristics of the sick group which they considered to be distinguishing features:

(1) They experienced considerably more early separation from
    parents, primarily through psychiatric hospitalisation of the
    mother.
(2) Teachers reported disturbing, aggressive behaviour at school.
(3) They showed a more rapid rate of recovery from momentary
    states of autonomic imbalance (measured by galvanic skin
    response, GSR).[1]
(4) Seventy per cent of the sick group had suffered from the effects
    of serious pregnancy and/or birth complications as babies.

Of interest too was the finding that high-risk subjects who did not

[1] Skin conductance of electricity can be measured by placing two electrodes on the palm. It
reflects the amount of sweating and has been used as a measure of arousal towards a presenting
stimulus.

experience a breakdown had fewer perinatal problems than the low-risk subjects. This suggested to the investigators that there may be a special interaction between genetic predisposition for schizophrenia, and pregnancy and delivery complications (Mednick *et al.*, 1981a). Perhaps the high-risk individual needed a trouble-free birth in order to stand a good chance of avoiding schizophrenia.

A further follow-up in 1972 collected more detailed diagnostic information. By this time ten of the 207 high-risk subjects had died, seven by suicide, two by accidental causes and one by a natural cause. None of the low-risk subjects had died. Thirteen of the high-risk subjects were diagnosed as schizophrenic. The investigators reported from a previous publication in which they had compared these thirteen subjects with twenty-nine borderline schizophrenics, thirty-four neurotics and twenty-three high-risk subjects with no mental illness. This enabled them once again to draw up a profile of those high-risk subjects who developed schizophrenia, which turned out to be similar to that reported at an earlier stage of the research. The thirteen children who developed schizophrenia could be characterised by the following factors: their birth had been relatively difficult (longer and more complicated than average); most of them had been separated from both parents and many placed in children's homes at a young age; they posed a disciplinary problem to their teachers; and some years earlier they had had a rapid autonomic nervous system (ANS) recovery rate. Furthermore, the high-risk children who developed the disorder could be distinguished from high-risk children who had so far shown no signs of developing the condition by the seriousness of the schizophrenic illness suffered by their mothers (as judged by the age at which their symptoms had begun).

However, there seemed to be important sex differences in the way these early factors related to the development of schizophrenia. The age at which the mother's illness had begun was the only factor directly related to the presence of schizophrenia in women. In men this factor was only related because of its association with separation. Separation, perinatal complications and ANS recovery responsiveness related to the development of schizophrenia in boys (Mednick *et al.*, 1981a). Behavioural precursors of schizophrenia included a poor emotional rapport in the psychiatric interview, and parental observations that he or she had been a passive baby, with a short attention span in childhood, and often impolite behaviour, while school reports often noted that the child was isolated, uneasy about criticism, easily upset, and disturbed the class (Parnas *et al.*, 1982).

Finally, evidence is accumulating that a person's emotional environment influences his or her likelihood of suffering an acute psychotic episode if he or she already has a history of schizophrenic disorder. If the person lives with a family member with whom he has an intense relationship, characterised by a high level of criticism and overinvolvement, his risk of relapse is much higher than it would be in a less intense atmosphere (Brown *et al.*, 1972; Leff and Vaughn, 1981). Not surprisingly, this finding has led to further speculation about the role of hostile, critical and overprotective parenting in the first onset of schizophrenia. However, despite some thought-provoking case studies collected by Leff and Vaughn (1985) which illustrate the sorts of unusual parent-child relationships which they have found, there is little good research to inform the debate. The findings of Doane *et al.* (1981) from their five-year follow-up of sixty-five disturbed (and therefore considered high-risk) adolescents provide some tentative indication that such abnormal parenting may have some causal significance, but the evidence is not that strong. They assessed both communication deviance and affective style at the first interview with families, that is, aspects such as disruptive speech, closure problems, unclear communication of ideas, and statements that were supportive, critical, guilt-inducing or intrusive. They found that the two measures did not separately hold any predictive value, but in combination they discriminated well between families in which a child developed some schizophrenic symptoms and those whose child remained free of such symptoms.

As these young people were already disturbed these factors cannot be claimed to have predated disturbed behaviour, but they did exist prior to the appearance of psychotic-like disorders. The investigators suggested that the combination of communication deviance and critical, intrusive or guilt-inducing affect from parents meant that their adolescent child had 'little recourse through communication with them for exploring, clarifying, or correcting his feelings of unworthiness, rejection, or isolation'.

These ideas are in some ways similar to one of the psychoanalytical theories of schizophrenia, popular in the 1960s, Bateson's 'double-bind' hypothesis. This also states that the individuals concerned must be in an intense relationship and that it is impossible or very difficult for the victim to 'escape from the field'. The bind arises when the speaker expresses two or more messages which are incompatible, at different levels of communication. For example, the subject's mother may be verbally expressing affection while her facial expression and movements convey contempt or a lack of concern. The individual is presented from commenting on the inconsistencies in that if he attempts to do so, he is met by condemnation that increases the confusing bind (Bateson *et al.*, 1956).

A wide range of organic and psychosocial differences between people who suffer from schizophrenia and a random sample of the general population have been identified. Yet the great mystery of schizophrenia remains – it is still unclear precisely what role, if any, such factors have had in bringing about the first onset of the disorder. Many of the differences identified predate the emergence of any specific schizophrenic symptoms. But this does not mean they caused them to appear. For instance, a child may inherit a predisposition to schizophrenia, which causes him to have certain childhood adjustment problems, which in turn bring about unusual family communication styles. This means that family and school problems may be common antecedents of schizophrenia, but have no causal role in bringing it about. Alternatively, it may only be when family relationships are poor that the inherited predisposition is likely to lead to schizophrenia. Do obstetric complications leave an invisible injury which later manifests itself in combination with a certain inherited characteristic as a particular vulnerability to schizophrenia? Or does a difficult birth seem to be associated with schizophrenia because it causes the mother to feel overprotective or guilty towards the child who started life so badly? In which case, it would be the mother's behaviour, rather than any brain damage, which had causal significance. These are just some of the many possible answers to this fascinating riddle.

Psychosocial factors in the course of schizophrenic disorder

The evidence on social factors related to the course of schizophrenic disorder is still the most valuable information available for prevention.

Once the disorder has developed, the impact of environmental circumstances on its course and outcome is relatively easily established: the difficult issue of reconstructing family relationships and other environmental circumstances as they existed before the appearance of symptoms is unnecessary. All that is needed is a reliable assessment of current circumstances. Two sets of findings in particular suggest preventive strategies that could considerably reduce the prevalence of acute psychotic episodes. Both relate to the social environment of the person with an established schizophrenic illness: while he is being treated for the disorder in hospital, and after he has been discharged into the community.

A study by Wing and Brown (1970) suggested that people with schizophrenia were likely to respond to understimulation by withdrawal and regression. Their controlled study showed that the social withdrawal and poverty of speech of chronic patients varied from one hospital to another according to the severity of ward restrictiveness, absence of personal belongings, and the length of time that patients were left to do nothing. On the other hand, overstimulation, especially in emotionally arousing circumstances, was likely to result in an acute exacerbation of symptoms. The latter finding arose from an observation by Brown and his colleagues (1966) that patients discharged to live alone or in a hostel often fared rather better than those who went to live with a spouse or parent. They went on to develop a method of rating family relationships from interviews in the relatives' home (the Camberwell Family Interview, Brown and Rutter, 1966). Interviews were tape-recorded so that a trained rater could play back the tape and rate the relatives on: critical comments, hostility, overinvolvement, warmth and positive remarks. The rater took account of the tone of voice as well as what was being said. Critical comments, hostility and overinvolvement, generally termed 'expressed emotion' (EE), on the part of the relative most closely associated with the patient have been shown to be related to risk of relapse (Brown et al., 1972; Vaughn and Leff, 1976).

Maintenance medication and a reduction of time spent in face-to-face contact with a high 'EE' relative was shown by these studies to reduce the risk associated with living in a high 'EE' home. This meant that there were essentially three variables which could affect risk of relapse: level of EE, level of contact, and maintenance medication. Brown and his colleagues (1972) studied 101 patients, Vaughn and Leff (1976), 128. Of those returning to a high EE home, 58 per cent and 51 per cent of these two samples relapsed within nine months. This compared to 16 per cent and 13 per cent of those going to live with low EE relatives. However, where the level of contact with the high EE relative was greater than thirty-five hours per week, risk of relapse rose to 79 per cent and 67 per cent of the

samples. If patients lived with a low EE relative, the major tran-
quillising drugs produced a relatively small reduction in relapse rate.
But for patients in high EE homes, the continued use of these drugs
reduced the relapse rate over a nine-month period among Brown
and his colleagues' sample by one third (66 per cent to 46 per cent),
and in Vaughn and Leff's sample, by about one half. As each of the
three variables seemed to be related to risk of relapse, it followed
that those living in high contact with high EE relatives and failing to
maintain prophylactic medication should be at greatest risk of relapse,
while those living with low EE relatives and continuing to take their
medication should have the lowest risk. Vaughn and Leff (1976)
found the relapse rate to be 92 per cent compared to 12 per cent
for patients falling into these two extreme groups over the same nine-
month period.

Furthermore, intervention programmes aiming to reduce the level
of expressed emotion among relatives high on this index, or alternatively to reduce their level of face-to-face contact, have shown that
relapse rates can be reduced in this way (e.g. Leff *et al.*, 1982;
1985; Falloon *et al.*, 1982; and see chapter 9). These findings add
considerable weight to the claims that emotional arousal is of causal
significance to relapse. Taken together, these studies provide
numerous practical indications for the management of schizophrenia.

Brown and Birley (1968) argued that people who have a history
of schizophrenia have a high sensitivity to their social environment
even when they have no apparent symptoms. This idea of an optimum
arousal level which may easily be upset by under- or overstimulating
conditions has also been put forward by Venables (1964). This means
that people who have suffered or are currently suffering from schizophrenia need to be able to withdraw from arousing circumstances,
but that the extreme understimulation which could sometimes be
found in an old-fashioned mental hospital should equally be avoided.
Patients in understimulating environments also show a high level of
arousal.

This information is potentially very valuable for those in a position
to help families to find the best ways of supporting the patient at
home in the process of rehabilitation. They could be taught, for
instance, that the patient may sometimes need to withdraw from
social contact with his or her family. This might help them to see
his lack of social responsiveness as a symptom of his illness and
something for which they should make allowances rather than as an

unfriendly act or a personal slight on their company. However, this kind of educational process needs to be carried out with extreme care. Information which places guilt for the patient's illness on the family might only serve to reinforce their overprotective and critical communication styles, which may have arisen in the first place for just this reason. Indeed, the widespread public belief in the role parents may have in causing adjustment problems in their children, and the guilt, shame and stigma associated with such views, may become circular. Warner (1985) points out that living with someone whose actions can be unpredictable and distressing, and whose emotional responses are unrewarding, is difficult enough. But with the reactions of society to the disturbed person and to his relatives, these problems may be sufficient in themselves to produce distorted patterns of family interaction. Birley and Hudson (1983) and Berkowitz and her colleagues (1984) have given sensitive descriptions of the ways in which the family might best be helped.

Not surprisingly, given the sensitivity to arousal, life events have also been found to play a role in bringing about an acute relapse. Brown and Birley (1968) found 46 per cent of their sample of schizophrenic patients to have experienced an independent life event (one unlikely to have been a consequence of the previous illness) in the three weeks before onset, compared to 14 per cent of a comparison group of factory and office workers in the three weeks prior to their interview. Paykel (1979) also reported an excess of life events in the six months before a patient's first admission for schizophrenia compared to a general population sample in New Haven. Unlike the situation for depression, however, the events implicated in schizophrenia will not necessarily be those which appear threatening or unfavourable. Exciting or arousing events like being promoted or winning a competition may have a similar effect (Brown and Birley, 1968). However, while it might seem that in high EE homes, people with schizophrenia would be particularly vulnerable to relapse after a life event, Leff and Vaughn (1980) failed to find an excess of events in the weeks preceding relapse for patients in high EE homes. In fact, nine of the ten patients experiencing a life event in the latter study were in low EE homes. They conclude that the onset or relapse of schizophrenia is associated either with high EE *or* with an independent life event. Both Brown and Birley (1968) and Leff and Vaughn (1980) found that life events tend to be concentrated in the three weeks before the onset of schizophrenic symptoms.

It is uncertain whether neuroleptic medication is protective against the effects of life events, although it is well accepted to be protective against high emotional arousal. However, it may be helpful to adjust the dose at the critical time. It may also be feasible to prepare patient and relatives for predictable events or even to avoid such situations altogether (Brown *et al.*, 1972).

A model of schizophrenia

The most well-recognised factor in the aetiology of schizophrenia is that a genetic vulnerability is inherited. Trauma at birth may also play some part in forming the newborn infant's predisposition to develop the disorder. One possible explanation of the condition is a dysfunction of the right hemisphere of the brain and an overcompensation by the left side. The person will have a high level of emotional arousal and be particularly sensitive to social influences which can affect arousal. Relapse of florid symptoms and possibly their first onset can be precipitated by stressful events. Relapse in the absence of a precipitating event is most likely to occur when the patient is living in a situation characterised by high expressed emotion between himself and a relative with whom he has a high degree of contact. Neuroleptic medication provides some kind of protective effect against relapse. Reducing the amount of time a patient spends in face-to-face contact with relatives with whom he lives in a 'high EE' environment, or changing their communication styles, will also be protective. The association of factors such as psychiatric illness of parent, marital disharmony, overprotectiveness and abnormal thinking and communication may or may not be relevant to onset or relapse, or may simply be another result of the same genetic consti-tution which produced a child vulnerable to schizophrenia. Equally probable is that the pre-schizophrenic child and the schizophrenic adult produced some of the abnormalities of the parents.

It is clear that, as with depression, a complex interactive multifac-torial model is needed to explain the cause and course of schizo-phrenia. As with depression, a range of factors may contribute to a person's vulnerability to the disorder, and other factors may act to precipitate its appearance. A range of social and environmental circumstances of the individual will determine the subsequent course and outcome of the illness. Strauss and Carpenter (1981) conceptual-ised the development of schizophrenia as essentially having four levels. The first stage is the prenatal and perinatal period when a person's genetic constitution is determined, birth trauma may occur, and the early mother-child bond established. What happens at this stage will determine the infant's predisposition to schizophrenia. The developmental stage follows, when maladaptive learning and abnormal family communication patterns may each perhaps contribute to the young person's vulnerability to schizophrenia. A number of factors may then precipitate a psychotic episode, including emotionally arousing events and a stressful environment. Finally, the course and outcome of the disorder will be affected by the same kinds of events and environment, and by certain treatment and rehabilitation measures. These not only include the now standard pharmacological treatments, but also the patterns of institutional care, and, Warner (1985) would argue, the broader social environment as it affects reintegration and the social role rehabilitation of the individual (including the labelling, stigma and social isolation which may occur).

Hirsch and Leff (1975) have also put together several possible models of schizophrenia. These might be combined with the formulation above and adapted as shown in Figure 5.1.

This model is complex, but is just the first step in explaining the development of schizophrenia. Little progress has been made in terms of developing a theory of the disorder which would provide greater understanding of how and why these factors relate to each other. The theories which have been advanced so far have not been adequately tested in empirical research so as to gain credibility. Nevertheless, the model does show that a good deal is now known about the illness, and this information provides both promising avenues for future research and implications for preventive intervention. The search for physiological, psychological, social, biochemical or other markers which will facilitate the identification of high-risk children with some accuracy needs to continue. Possible research approaches include following up infants experiencing some perinatal trauma who also have a close biological relative with schizophrenia in the hopes of identifying other indicators of risk. Several longitudinal studies of this nature are already under way (e.g. Wrede et al., 1981).

Until further progress has been made to facilitate the identification of people at risk of schizophrenia, there is not a firm basis for large-scale intervention programmes. However, even at this stage, much might be learned from some experimental intervention trials, both

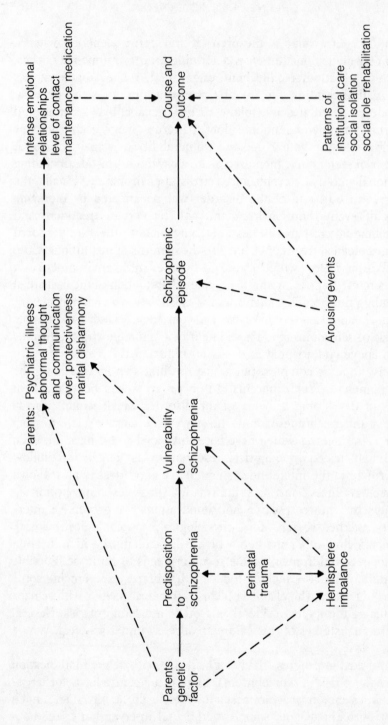

Figure 5.1 Schematic representation of factors suggested to be implicated in the development of schizophrenia

about aetiology and prevention. Perhaps, for instance, educational programmes for parents of disabled or ill children might be evaluated to see if reducing any over-involved or overcritical parenting styles reduces the child's later risk of schizophrenia. Families where there is both a record of schizophrenia and where the index child was born after a particularly long or difficult labour would be particularly suitable targets.

In terms of preventing relapse among people with an established schizophrenic illness, a concern for the social environment to which they return needs to become as much a part of standard procedures as is the administration of maintenance medication. The relatives of schizophrenic patients should routinely be involved in treatment programmes (Leff, 1985). Where the home environment seems to be unsupportive in as much as it is highly arousing, strategies to increase the social distance in key relationships, or to modify their ways of interacting, would be helpful. Daytime employment, sheltered work, or a place at a day centre or day hospital may be one answer, or removal to a hostel or group home. Adherence to the maintenance drugs regime will nearly always be helpful to people treated for schizophrenia in the process of rehabilitation, but is likely to be especially important for those remaining in living circumstances that are far from ideal. Monitoring and encouraging drug maintenance is largely an administrative task which requires flexible hospital and clinic opening times, a local register of patients needing regular treatment, and for social and clinical services to maintain a constant link to ensure continuous monitoring (Freeman, 1978).

Finally, for those people with a family member with schizophrenia whose distress and disturbed behaviour may dramatically affect them, there must also be preventive implications for themselves in their involvement in the treatment programme. Marjorie Wallace (1985) has collected accounts from seventy-five families of schizophrenic sufferers from all over the country, who paint a harrowing tale of fear, loss and powerlessness as they watch a member of their family gradually disintegrate. Often a son or daughter will have been on the brink of a promising career when they developed their first symptoms. One-third of sufferers will never experience a second episode, but for the rest it may be a lifetime's struggle against repeated attacks, each one taking its toll. It seems likely that for a parent or spouse, the experience may well be comparable to the sorts of events and difficulties implicated in depression. For their own sakes, as well as the patient's, they need information about the condition. They need to understand the importance of the regular drug treatment, and they need to be supported in their efforts to deal with their own guilt, depression and daily stress of living with a person with schizophrenia. They can be helped to relate to the disturbed individual in the most supportive manner (Leff *et al.*, 1982), and to help him develop positive skills (Falloon *et al.*, 1982). But they also need to have their own anxieties answered (for example, about side-effects of the drugs), and, in dealing with a severe and recurring disorder, they need periodic relief from their caring responsibility, advice on financial supplements available and a knowledge of good ways of coping with difficult behaviour on the part of their disturbed relative.

6
Prevention in childhood

It has long been assumed that the origins of many adult disorders lie somewhere in childhood or earlier events. Whether a biological or psychosocial perspective has been taken, events of aetiological significance have been sought in the individual's formative stages, from fertilisation and intrauterine development, to parent-child relationships in early and middle childhood. However, the preceding chapters have shown just how many possible mediating processes may explain the apparent link between childhood risk factors and adult disorder. Any factor found to occur more often than would be expected by chance in the childhood histories of adult psychiatric cases could be linked to disorder in at least three ways.

Firstly, the antecedent factor may be a direct cause of childhood psychiatric disturbance which has a continuous of intermittent course into adulthood. The same kinds of symptom may be present throughout, or the disorder may manifest itself in different forms at different life stages, perhaps as conduct disorder or delinquency in childhood, but in adulthood as alcoholism or even schizophrenia. Secondly, there may be a continuity of psychiatric problems only if the risk factor also persists. Perhaps a lack of supportive parent-child relationship is associated with childhood problems, but only if the person continues to lack a close supportive relationship in later life will psychiatric problems continue or recur. Thirdly, the factor may not result in any significant childhood disturbance, but may produce disorder in later life as other risk factors accumulate. For instance, maternal psychiatric disorder may have a deleterious effect on the mother-child relationship not serious enough to produce a disorder in the child, but may also set in motion a chain of other, more powerful adverse events. The child may be separated from his mother while she receives treatment, her marriage may collapse and the family break up, and subsequent living circumstances may be stressful and socially deprived. Any one, or a combination of all these events may turn out to have key importance in the later development of disorder.

There are, undoubtedly, some aetiological links between early life experiences, events in later childhood and adolescence, and circumstances in adult life. In recent decades, considerable progress has been made in identifying personal and social factors which can be damaging or protective, and some of the complex interrelationships between events and circumstances that contribute to psychiatric risk (Rutter, 1985). Although our understanding is far from complete, there are many valuable pointers to the elements likely to be necessary in effective prevention. In this chapter, some of the evidence will be reviewed which sheds some light on three questions. What do we know about the determinants of childhood disorder? Under what circumstances does childhood disorder continue into adulthood? And what do we know about childhood determinants of adult disorder which might be amenable to preventive intervention? The following does not attempt to be a comprehensive review of the aetiology of childhood disorder, but to reveal some of the important factors which will have to be considered in conceptualising prevention through intervention with children.

Determinants of childhood disorder

Emotional and conduct disorders are the most frequently encountered psychiatric disturbances of childhood. And as Wolff (1983a, p. 37) points out, 'despite important constitutional, social and medical disadvantages which often contribute to their genesis, the disorders themselves are most helpfully explained on the basis of psychological mechanisms.'

Children with conduct disorder behave in a way seen as troublesome to others and do not conform to expected social norms. They may fight with other children, be difficult for their parents and teachers to control, or steal. Their disobedience may include running away from home, disruptive classroom behaviour at school, precocious indulgence in alcohol or addictive substances, and sexual promiscuity (Shaffer, 1983, p. 9). Three out of four will be male, and one in three doing poorly in their schoolwork. Their parents will often have marital problems (Rutter *et al.*, 1970). Children with

emotional problems may, for instance, be excessively afraid of stran-
gers or of separating from their parents. They may be unduly withdrawn or subdued. They are equally likely to be male or female and
there is no characteristic family disturbance (Rutter *et al.*, 1970).
Children and adolescents may often have a combination of conduct
and emotional problems. There are other, less common disturbances
in childhood and adolescence, including childhood psychosis, the
hyperkinetic syndrome and anorexia nervosa.

Of course, shyness, fears, depression of mood, disobedience,
fighting, stealing and temper tantrums are often part of ordinary day-
to-day behaviour. It is only when the frequency and magnitude of
each behaviour is sufficiently marked and sufficiently prolonged to
impede the child himself in his daily life or cause distress to his
family or community that it can be defined as disorder (Rutter *et al.*,
1970).

In looking for causal explanations of disorder, Wolff (1983a) argues
that both scientific and subjective explanations are needed. This is
because in children, even more than in adults, pathological behaviour
is the outcome of an interactional process. Age is the most obvious
factor that will change the subjective interpretation of events. Young
children will often, for instance, feel a sense of responsibility for
adverse events in which they in fact had no role at all, and hence
experience a good deal of anxiety. Children may also react to deprivation or lack of attention by showing difficult or aggressive behaviour. If interpreted by the parent as hostile and rejecting behaviour,
and responded to in turn by punishment and rejection, a mutually
reinforcing pattern of hostile interaction may begin.

A large number of factors have been identified as contributing to
the development of childhood psychiatric disorder in some way.

(i) Age

The child's developing cognitive capacities mean that events which
at one age produce little or no anxiety may, at another, be extremely
distressing. Mother-child separation at four months of age may not
be too disturbing, as the child will not yet have formed a lasting
selective attachment to her. The reasons for a separation and its
temporary nature can be explained to a ten-year-old child, so that
anxiety can again be minimised. But at age two or three years, a

threat of loss is understood, but the reasons for the separation and its temporary nature may not be.

From three years onwards, children can experience a fear of injury, and illness and accidents may generate excessive anxiety (Wolff, 1983a). Fears, phobias and nightmares are also at their height at ages three to five. At around six years of age, the child enters a wider social group and can perceive stigma, and experience a loss of self-esteem (Wolff, 1983a). He may then become fully aware of any physical, social or educational disadvantages he possesses.

(ii) Sex

Boys are constitutionally more predisposed to the development of aggressive behaviour than are girls (Wolff, 1983a). There may also be some sex-linked predisposition to developmental disorders such as enuresis, encopresis and retarded reading as these tend to occur more often in boys than girls. Boys also seem to suffer more than girls when family discord and family disruption occur. There are several possible interactive processes to explain these findings. There has been some suggestion that parents are more likely to argue in front of their sons than their daughters; that a disturbed parent is more likely to pick on a son than a daughter; and that mothers may transfer negative experiences with their husband into negative expectations of their sons. Furthermore children tend to identify with the parent of the same sex. Fathers are more often aggressive and also are more often absent from the home. If the mother denigrates her husband, it is more likely that a boy will become particularly anxious (Wolff, 1983b).

(iii) Temperament

A longitudinal study by Thomas and Chess (1977) of 141 children from predominantly middle-class homes in New York showed a marked continuity of temperamental disposition. The mothers had been interviewed periodically since the children were two or three months old about such characteristics as the child's activity level, adaptability, distractability, persistence and quality of mood. Active children tended to have been active, difficult babies, and passive children withdrawn babies, low in persistence. Such characteristics inevitably help to shape parent reactions, which in turn affect the child's adjustment. For instance, it has been noted that when 'parents are depressed and irritable they do not take it out on all their children to the same extent: often one is more or less scapegoated. The target child tends to be the temperamentally difficult one' (Rutter, 1979a, p. 57).

(iv) Brain damage

Rutter (1977) has shown that brain-damaged children are at greater risk of psychiatric disorder than undamaged children, possibly due more to abnormal brain activity rather than to a straightforward loss of brain function. The crucial cognitive effects of damage are due to both general intellectual impairment and specific reading retardation. However, some of the increased risk will be caused indirectly through the stigma associated with scholastic failure, the increased likelihood of difficult temperamental characteristics, and scapegoating or over-protection on the part of his or her parents. If the condition requires frequent hospital admissions and a restriction of physical activity, further adverse effects may occur.

(v) Low intelligence, educational retardation

The surveys by Rutter and his colleagues in the Isle of Wight revealed a high correlation between psychiatric disturbance and intellectual retardation (Rutter et al., 1970). Retarded children were over three times as likely to be disturbed as children in the comparison group (23 per cent versus 7 per cent). Furthermore, one-third of severely retarded readers had conduct disorders. The high level of social maladjustment among children attending schools for the moderately educationally retarded has also been well documented. Newton and Robinson (1982) found half of the sixteen-year-olds in four inner London ESN(M) schools to be maladjusted, as rated by the Bristol Social Adjustment Scales, while in South Wales, Chazan (1964) reported a similar proportion: 50 per cent of the boys, 32 per cent of the girls.

(vi) Schooling

The Isle of Wight and London surveys (Rutter et al. 1975a; 1975b) found markedly differing rates of behaviour problems and reading difficulties between one primary school and another. The children were followed up some four years later at secondary schools so that the possibility could be considered that such differences were attributable to initial differences in their ability and adjustment rather than being caused by the schools (Rutter *et al.*, 1979). Differences between schools remained, and were not explicable in terms of differences in intake, family characteristics or primary school attended. It was concluded that good schools can, and do, exert an important protective effect against behavioural disturbance. The quality of the schools as social institutions appeared to be more important than their size, administration, or the age of the buildings. A 'good' school had a balanced intake of ability levels, widespread opportunity for pupil participation and individual responsibility, good classroom management and discipline, often an academic emphasis, and a wide use of rewards and incentives. A preponderance of low-ability children, or of disadvantaged or ethnic minority children, was associated with raised delinquency rates.

As described in chapter 4, Quinton and Rutter (1983) found that positive school experiences appeared to help foster planning skills in girls brought up in care. In late adolescence and young adulthood, planning skills were in turn related to social functioning and parenting behaviour. A positive experience of school was not only a reflection of examination success, but may also have resulted from good relationships with peers or a positive memory of several other aspects of school life. It seemed that for girls lacking a source of self-esteem in their home lives, schools could be particularly important in this respect.

(vii) Parental mental illness, marital discord, family break-up

These three factors must be considered together because it seems that both parental mental illness and parental separation or divorce may have a particularly damaging effect on the children if they are associated with prolonged overt marital discord, especially where the child becomes directly involved. Rutter (1979a) quotes research evidence to show that both maternal psychiatric disorder and paternal criminality are associated with disturbed behaviour in the children. Sons of aggressive, sociopathic fathers are particularly prone to conduct disorder (Robins, 1966). High rates of depression among mothers of young children and a strong association between maternal depression and disturbance in the children have been found by

Richman (1978) and Crook and Wolkind (1983). Similarly, Pound and her colleagues (1985) found that a long history of depressive illness in a mother, or a combination of depression and personality problems, was associated with problems (especially of sleeping) in her children. A catalogue of past and present social difficulties was associated with the mothers' depression. They argue, however, that marital discord (common among the depressed sample) added to, rather than was responsible for, the effects of maternal depression on the child.

A constellation of social difficulties has also been found to characterise parents who severely physically abuse their children. Baldwin (1977) traced all child victims of severe abuse (damage on the scale of multiple fractures, internal injuries, brain damage and death) who were under the age of five years and living in North East Wiltshire over an eight-year period. Fathers or father surrogates were often unemployed, families moved home frequently, father figures changed or left the family home often, mothers were very young (average age twenty-one years) but already had an average of three children. The parent figures as a group showed gross excesses of psychiatric disturbance, physical illness and disability, and criminality, and the abusing parent had often been subjected to physical or mental abuse or neglect in their own childhood. Severe abuse was viewed by Baldwin as an outcome of overwhelming stress in families profoundly disabled by illness, personality disorder, inadequacy or incompetence. Similarly, Delozier (1982) has described the histories of eighteen 'typical' abusing mothers, which show that their childhood contained much more by way of threat of abandonment and harm than that of a comparison group of mothers.

Parental divorce has often been assumed to have deleterious effects on children. However, it is more likely that the marital conflict which precedes the separation and the stressful events which follow it are the real sources of difficulty. Hetherington (1979) found that if marital separation led to a cessation of hostilities and conflict, this seemed somewhat less damaging for children than remaining in a discordant, unhappy, but intact home.

Hetherington (1979) charts the common problems which accompany divorce. For instance, mothers often experience downward economic mobility as income from the father drops, sometimes requiring moving to more modest housing, which in turn may involve loss of friends, neighbours and a familiar educational system.

Mothers caring for their children on their own may need to find outside employment, and the strain of the dual role may result in a chaotic lifestyle where the children get less attention, household chores remain undone and mealtimes and bedtimes become erratic. In the first twelve months marital conflict present before the divorce often increases, and parents become inconsistent, less affectionate, and lacking in control over their children. Following this period, parenting usually improves again, and most children readjust. Vital to this readjustment, however, is a continued supportive relationship with the parent with whom the children live, and the involvement of the spouse in supporting the children and the divorced partner in their parenting role (Hetherington, 1979). In the long term, the quality of life which the divorced or remarried family make for themselves becomes the most important factor in determining whether any disturbed behaviour persists (Wallerstein, 1984).

In a stressful home environment, whether the difficulties are due to parental mental illness or family discord, it seems that a good relationship with one parent (or both parents), characterised by a high level of warmth and the absence of severe criticism, is protective. Only a quarter of children with a good relationship and living in a discordant home showed a conduct disorder in a study reported by Rutter (1979a), compared to three-quarters of those lacking such a relationship. Furthermore, a longitudinal study which charted the progress of children in discordant homes, also reported by Rutter, documented the marked reduction in psychiatric risk which followed a substantial improvement in the home environment, when compared to the progress of children remaining in unhappy, quarrelsome homes.

(viii) Mother-child separation

The influential work of John Bowlby has led many people to believe that any kind of mother-child separation during the first few years of a child's life should be avoided. He showed that many young children separated from their mothers for admissions to hospital or a residential nursery experienced an acute stress reaction followed by disturbing behaviour lasting many months. Bowlby argued that this was a direct consequence of the damaging effect of the separation on the emotional bond between mother and child (Bowlby, 1951; 1973). Rutter (1981) argued, however, that it is the circumstances surrounding any separation which are crucial, and that separation *per se* is not necessarily harmful.

Nevertheless, children between the ages of six months and three and a half years appear to be often adversely affected by hospital admissions lasting longer than one week, or by repeated admissions. Douglas (1975) showed from a long-term follow-up of a birth cohort of over 5,000 children that such admissions were associated with troublesome behaviour at school, and to low reading scores at age fifteen years. Quinton and Rutter (1976) replicated this finding, and were able to show that disorder resulting from hospital admission was not explicable in terms of other medical factors such as persisting disability or low birth weight. However, children from unhappy, disrupted or deprived homes were most likely to be damaged by the experience. Approximately 4 per cent of the general population experience multiple hospital admissions in childhood, and two-fifths of these are likely to show later disturbance. The overall numbers involved are therefore not insubstantial.

In the absence of adverse circumstances, however, it seems that most short-term parent-child separations will not usually be associated with any psychiatric risk. Children are not at increased psychiatric risk if their mother goes out to work, for instance, providing the alternative day care arrangements are of good quality, ensuring continuity of caretaking, adequate love and attention and opportunity for play and conversation. Indeed, the findings of Brown and Harris (1978) suggest that a job outside the home may in certain circumstances help to maintain a mother's mental health, in which case it may be beneficial to her relationships with her children. However, if the timing of the mother starting work coincides with other disturbing events such as death of the father, it may well be interpreted as a threatening event and lead to some distress.

While short-term separation of parent and child under favourable circumstances is unlikely to be damaging to the child, long-term separations can have more serious effects, particularly when they occur in the first three to four years of the child's life. Children cared for by grandmothers or foster mothers during their first three or four years often have great difficulty when they return to live with their natural parents or a new step-parent. Child psychiatrists see many emotionally and behaviourally disordered children with such experiences (Wolff, 1983a).

Children brought up in community homes are also over-represented among psychiatric clinic attenders. Their parenting experiences prior to reception into care is thought to contribute to their high rate of psychiatric disorder (Rutter, 1981). When children have been taken into care at a very early age, and have lived in institutions until after their third birthday, or have experienced several changes of foster mother during this time, they have sometimes failed to form any secure affectional bond or attachment. These circumstances have been linked with a raised probability that the child will later develop a syndrome labelled 'affectionless psychopathy' (Rutter, 1981; Wolkind, 1974). This personality disorder is characterised by a lack of guilt and an inability to keep rules or form lasting relationships. Evidence in this area has led to the conclusion that institutions are not capable of providing adequate parenting for the very young child and to the statement by the Royal College of Psychiatrists (1983) to the Standing Committee on Children in Care in Britain that no child under the age of three years should ever be placed in a residential nursery.

(ix) Bereavement

Raphael (1982) provides qualitative descriptions of the experiences of thirty-five children aged between two and eight years in twenty families in which either the mother or father had died in the previous two to eight weeks. She documents the considerable difficulties involved for researchers in approaching bereaved families and countering the disapproval of many outside agencies. Those families in which a parent died from an illness known in advance to be terminal seemed to be better able to respond to the needs of their children, and to prepare them for the loss with information and emotional support. Sudden, unexpected deaths were found to present particular difficulty to the bereaved parent in communicating events and supporting the reaction of his or her children. Children were often given confusing information, not taken to the funeral and generally left with a poor understanding of the finality of the event. Raphael also suggests that bereaved parents who felt particularly unsupported themselves, lacking contact with the grandparents, for instance, were especially likely to be oblivious to, or deny, their children's needs at this time. These circumstances (unexpectedness and lack of a supportive network) have been linked to a raised probability of disturbed conduct and emotional disorder among young children following bereavement. Once again it seems that the consequences of the death on family life, rather than the direct effects of the loss, may be crucial. Often the surviving parent becomes depressed, the family may break up and there may be social and economic privation (Parkes, 1972). However, research on parental death in childhood at the time of the loss is sparse.

(x) Interactive processes

From this brief examination of some of the factors which can affect childhood psychiatric risk, it is apparent for each one of the examples that they are relevant only if certain other conditions prevail. Many traumatic events may be overcome without lasting damage if, for instance, the child has a continuous, warm, secure relationship with one parent or parent-substitute. Accidental death of a child's twin brother may be highly disturbing at five years, but have much less impact at five months. An alcoholic father may not be as disturbing to the temperamentally easy daughter who is seldom the target of her father's aggressive outbursts, while her more difficult brother may be regularly physically and emotionally battered. One short hospital stay may cause minimal difficulties in adjustment to a child returning to a happy home life. Another child, repeatedly admitted for treatment, or whose home life preceding and following his hospital stay is characterised by family discord, may be adversely affected by the experience.

It seems that, to a certain extent, the effects of stress are cumulative, but not in any straightforward additive way. The indications are that the existence of one difficulty increases the probability that other stresses will also occur. Children with difficult or disadvantaged home circumstances are more often admitted to hospital and residential care than other children. A child whose mother has just started full-time employment may only be likely to be disturbed by this event if he has also recently lost his father. Yet it is in precisely this sort of situation that a woman who has hitherto chosen to stay at home with her children may need to seek work.

Such patterns of stress may be so much more damaging than the sum of their separate effects because their co-existence leads to a different attribution of meaning to them on the part of the child. A good relationship with one parent may, for example, be protective against the effects of mental illness in the other parent, if it enables the child to see the ill parent's behaviour for what it is, and not as a rejection of the child or caused by the child. In fact, many childhood difficulties may not, in isolation, raise psychiatric risk at all. A child who is enabled to cope well with a parent's illness, say, may well become *more* competent and resilient to adversity in the future.

(xi) Implications for prevention

Some risk factors in childhood may be amenable to prevention. Examples include the prevention of brain damage through: adequate perinatal care; prompt treatment of *status epilepticus*; the reduction of child abuse; and accident prevention (particularly road accidents). Immunisation for teenage girls against rubella also reduces the chance that pregnant women will catch and transmit the infection to their unborn children, with possible resultant brain damage; and biochemical screening of pregnant women to detect phenylketonuria enables the condition to be treated promptly in the newborn infant (Graham, 1977). Treatment of parental mental illnesses may also be seen as potential preventive approaches for childhood disturbance, as can efforts to help disadvantaged families find ways of resolving their multiple problems, and strategies to reduce overt marital discord. In this respect, it would seem to be more important that family relationships improve, whether or not husband and wife remain together, rather than urging parents to 'stick it out for the sake of the children' in unhappy marriages. Many workers in Britain have argued in favour of special family courts for divorcing families, and for divorce conciliation services, to help couples who wish to separate do so as amicably as possible (see for example, Parkinson, 1982).

The public concern and media coverage of cases of severe child abuse has produced a plethora of professional reviews suggesting ways victims can more rapidly be ascertained and recommendations for action when child abuse is suspected (DHSS, 1974). If one child in a family is maltreated, others in the same family are at high risk. Baldwin (1977) found that if the eldest child was abused, the likelihood that the second eldest would be abused was 78 per cent. If the two eldest were abused, 64 per cent of the third eldest were too. In cases of abuse as severe as those assessed by Baldwin, the ascertainment of one child should enable early ascertainment of abuse to subsequent children.

When the risk factor cannot be eradicated, or the stressful experience avoided, an alternative approach to prevention is to focus attention instead on the child's resources for coping with the problem. Perhaps he can be helped to interpret the events as less threatening. If a child must face a prolonged period of hospitalisation, say, he could relatively easily be prepared in advance with information about what will take place, and allowed to experience graded separations in happy circumstances, such as overnight stays with friends. In hospital, the parents can be enabled to spend as much time as they wish with their sick child, and efforts can be made to keep to the child's familiar routines (Rutter, 1979b). Or if an adult hospital patient with young children is known to be terminally ill, it should be possible to provide some kind of support for the spouse and the children in preparation for their loss, in order that they may work through their grief and come to terms with their new situation.

However, for most pre-school children, their sense of meaning and their self-esteem derive primarily from their interactions with their mothers. Yet multiple disadvantages are common in young families. Maternal depression, poverty and other social difficulties are highest among this section of the population, and these hazards are associated with a high rate of child disturbance. Few women are prepared for the difficulties of running a home and bringing up young children. Their knowledge is likely to be based on their memories of their own parenting. Since the traditional extended family network seems to be playing less and less of a role in supporting the young parent there may well be a need to substitute this source of information, advice and emotional support. Parenting education might begin in schools and continue over the first few years of married life (Pound et al., 1985). Postnatal support groups and mother and child playgroups are possible sources of companionship and parent education. More than specific child management skills, parents need to be aware of the level of understanding of their child, his anxieties, frustrations and emotional needs. Parents of low birth weight or handicapped children also need to be encouraged to avoid becoming overprotective, and communicating their anxieties to their children (Graham, 1977).

From the age of five years, schools may play a protective role. The findings of Rutter and his colleagues on the social structure of schools speak for themselves (see above). It also seems that it might be helpful if teachers were aware of those among their pupils with particularly unsupportive home lives, that is, with few sources outside school from which they might derive a sense of their own value. They might make special efforts for these children to maximise the chances that they will have some sort of positive experience in their school lives. It might be success on the sports field or in drama, a role as form captain, or enjoyable extra-curricular events. And finally, those children with reading difficulties need to be provided with remedial programmes as early as possible, and concerted efforts need to be made to minimise the sense of stigma they might experience because of their intellectual or physical disadvantage.

Does childhood disorder continue into adulthood?

Although a well-respected body of opinion favours the belief that an enduring emotional attachment between mother and baby develops during the infant's first year of life and the quality and strength of this bond is of paramount importance to the individual's future social and emotional development (Bowlby, 1951; Rutter, 1981), there is a surprising lack of research which has succeeded in demonstrating a continuity in the development of psychopathology. Efforts to chart continuities in maladjustment almost invariably fail to find more than a small relationship between early attachment or infant behaviour and later emotional or behavioural adjustment, and although very early relationships and behaviour are seen to be very important, most researchers aiming to demonstrate this fact end by concluding that discontinuity rather than continuity is the rule (e.g. Lewis *et al.*, 1984; Fischer *et al.*, 1984). Inevitably they argue that life stress events and family demographic variables are also important, and it may be the failure of much research to take these variables into account (and probably the problems of doing so) which explains why a stronger relationship between early attachment and behaviour and later adjustment is not found.

There is very little evidence, either, that young children with emotional disorders (anxiety, fear, depression) are more likely to suffer psychiatric disorders in adulthood than their more well-adjusted peers. However, there does seem to be some consensus of opinion and parallel findings to demonstrate continuity in the area of disorders of conduct (Robins, 1966; Rutter and Madge, 1976). Of course, one of the main difficulties in this kind of research lies in the collection of accurate information about events and experiences over a period of twenty years or more. If adults are asked about their childhood, it seems highly likely that their memories will have become distorted or lost over the years, and that they will be coloured by the person's present mood state, particularly by the existence of any psychiatric disorder. Hence a depressed person may well remember their childhood as considerably less happy than they would have done if asked the same questions before the onset of their current depressive symptoms. The ideal source of information is therefore that collected prospectively, that is, from subjects in their childhood who are then followed up and re-interviewed many years later.

For this reason, the study by Robins (1966) is probably still one of the best sources of descriptive evidence. Robins came across the intact records of a child guidance clinic in St Louis, of children who had been in trouble between 1924 and 1929. She successfully traced over 90 per cent of these individuals some thirty years later, and collected information about them from interviews and records, including assessments by psychiatrists on the presence of psychiatric disturbance. Altogether she followed up 345 white American children who had been referred to the child guidance clinic for anti-social behaviour, 130 other referrals and 100 individuals who had attended neighbouring elementary schools who had not been referred for any specialist help, and who therefore provided a comparison group.

Her most well-known finding was that the

> prognosis for children referred for anti-social behaviour is much less promising than that for children referred to child guidance units for other reasons. For anti-social boys – the risk of future arrests was 71 per cent . . . . For anti-social girls – the risk of divorce was 70 per cent and for boys – 50 per cent. Half the men and one-third of the women were heavy drinkers. Children with other kinds of referrals are more like the comparison school children at follow up – less of a problem both to society and to themselves.

She went on to say that

> it would follow from these findings that the children currently being referred to clinics for anti-social behaviour are the group for whom successful intervention is the more urgently needed, to prevent personal misery for them as adults, for their spouses and children, and for the persons whom they will rob or swindle.

The former clinic patients with anti-social behaviour were considerably more often diagnosed by the research psychiatrists as having a
sociopathic personality than were the comparison group. They were
also slightly more often diagnosed as suffering from alcoholism,
schizophrenia, hysteria and chronic brain syndrome. They did not
have a higher rate of manic depressive illness or anxiety neurosis. As
well as being powerful predictors of sociopathy, anti-social symptoms
were also better predictors than non-anti-social symptoms of hysteria
and alcoholism. In fact, many of the non-anti-social symptoms in
childhood seemed completely unrelated to adult psychiatric status.
For example, children who were fearful, withdrawn, shy, had tics,
were hypersensitive, had speech defects, insomnia, nightmares or
temper tantrums were no more likely to have psychiatric disorders
as adults than those lacking such traits in childhood.

The anti-social childhood behaviours which were found to be
significantly associated with adult sociopathy were: pathological lying,
lack of guilt, sexual perversion, impulsiveness, truanting, being a
runaway, physical aggression, a poor employment record, premarital
intercourse, theft, incorrigibility, staying out late, having 'bad' associates and recklessness. The presence of six or more of these factors
showed the strongest relationship with sociopathy, and their
frequency and seriousness also increased the relationship. But as
Robins points out in a later paper, a wide variety of anti-social
childhood behaviour predicts a wide variety of adult deviant behaviour, rather than, as some have claimed, particular behaviour being
predictive of specific offences (e.g. conduct disorder predicting property but not person offences). Three of the studies in which she has
been involved – that described here, a follow-up of normal young
black men, and a follow-up of Vietnam veterans – have supported
her contention that deviant behaviour of various types in childhood
or adolescence forms a syndrome which tends to continue in about
half the cases to adulthood. Thus, conduct disorder in childhood
indicates a high probability that a person will be arrested for a
criminal offence in adulthood, but does not predict the type of arrest
(Robins and Ratcliff, 1980).

Robins argued that disturbed behaviour in fathers tended to lead
to similar disturbances in their children, particularly their sons, as it
was a much better predictor of conduct disorders in the children
than was the behaviour of the mother or siblings. The relationship
was strongest where the father showed a wide range of disturbed

behaviour: excessive drinking, desertion, arrests, failure to support the family and a tendency to change jobs frequently, with long spells of unemployment. This was also thought to explain, at least partly, the high rate of conduct disorder among children in low socio-economic groups with discordant home backgrounds.

This raises another major problem in studying continuities in pathology, that of disentangling continuity of disorder from the continuity of causal social stressors. For instance, childhood conduct disorder may often lead to anti-social behaviour in adulthood, but this may reflect either the continuity of the disorder *or* the different effects of the same social stress acting first upon a child and later upon an adult (Graham, 1983). The assumption which seems to prevail in the literature on conduct disorder is that certain disordered personality characteristics are formed which tend to continue, although the data on continuities in adverse social conditions which would confirm this assumption is by and large absent. However, the implication is that intervention should focus on the prevention or early treatment of the disorder. Robins suggests that early identification of disorder should be possible through the school system, as most of her sample were already in obvious social difficulties before the age of ten years. As lack of discipline at home had been found to be important to later sociopathy, she recommended improved discipline at school for such at-risk youngsters: a more vigorous role in preventing truancy, supervision for completion of assignments, controlled use of leisure time and so on. Judicial action and institutionalisation were not recommended, as such action seemed to be associated with a higher rate of later sociopathic behaviour among her sample.

If a good deal of conduct disorder could be prevented or successfully treated in childhood, it would seem that such intervention should have considerable impact on the prevalence of personality disorder and sociopathic behaviour among adults. Success would, however, be less important to the prevention of disorders seen and treated by adult psychiatrists than to the problems dealt with by the criminal justice system. These sorts of childhood problems are only weakly linked to adult schizophrenia and alcoholism, and completely unrelated to manic depressive illness or anxiety neurosis.

Modifying early childhood experiences as a preventive intervention in adult disorder

In chapters 4 and 5, a range of childhood and early adult experiences were described which probably have some causal importance in depression and schizophrenia. Being brought up in an institution or by neglectful parents, a pregnancy, early marriage, and showing poor planning skills were considered to have a causal role in adult depression. Perinatal complications among babies born with an inherited predisposition towards schizophrenia may be implicated in the later manifestation of this disorder.

Some of these factors can be found in the descriptions provided by Robins (1966) of the childhood histories of the child guidance patients who later developed psychiatric problems. Although the study was primarily concerned with the continuity of anti-social behaviour, there were also twenty-nine men found to have alcoholism, twenty-three men diagnosed as schizophrenic, twenty women described as 'hysterics' and thirty-two male and thirty female 'other neurotics' who were predominantly either undiagnosed or anxiety states. Many of the same factors seem also to have occurred in the childhood histories of adults developing different disorders, suggesting that, as illustrated by Figure 3.1 (page 36), in different combinations the same factors may play an aetiological role in different disorders. For instance, apart from the group labelled 'other neurotics', a high rate of broken homes was characteristic of the whole group of adults with disorders when compared to child guidance patients found to be well as adults. Furthermore, an abundant sexual experience was common in childhood among the women described as having hysterical or sociopathic disorders, and strikingly inadequate discipline had been a feature of their homes.

In fact, over 80 per cent of the women with hysterical or sociopathic disorders had, as children, lived away from both natural parents at some time, and over a third of the men diagnosed in adulthood as schizophrenic had been taken into care during childhood. Only the 'other neurotic' group were indistinguishable as children from those who grew up to be well; if anything, their home lives were slightly more adequate than those of the comparison group.

What are the practical implications of following these pointers?

(i) Perinatal complications, parental mental illness, parental overconcern

There is a distinct possibility that perinatal trauma interacts in some way with an inherited predisposition towards schizophrenia to increase psychiatric risk. The children of women with schizophrenia followed up by Mednick and his colleagues (1981a) who eventually developed schizophrenia were more likely to have had perinatal complications than those who had had a non-traumatic birth. Further, Cutting (1985) cites research evidence which shows that in monozygotic twins discordant for schizophrenia, it is the identical twin experiencing the more complicated birth who is more likely to develop schizophrenia. This suggests that it may be beneficial to provide more intensive antenatal care for pregnant women with a history of schizophrenia, and to be particularly cautious in the management of their deliveries.

Overinvolvement by close relatives seems to be implicated in relapse of an established schizophrenic illness. But as yet no feature of parenting has been convincingly established as being a causal factor in the first onset of the disorder despite observations by numerous investigators that parent-child relationships are often atypical in a number of ways. Even without evidence of a causal role in schizophrenia, the reduction of overprotective parenting may be seen to be a valuable preventive strategy for other psychiatric problems. Child psychiatrists provide many clinical accounts of the high level of overprotection among parents of children with emotional disorders, especially if such children have a physical handicap or illness or other evidence of fragility (Graham, 1977). It seems likely that just as extremes of neglect may have long-term deleterious consequences, so may overprotection. Clinicians could perhaps reduce the transmission of anxiety to disabled or ill children by more positive reassurance and support to their parents, and by helping parents whose children have recovered from complications at birth to realise that they are no longer in any danger and can be treated like other children. Mutual aid groups and health visitors may also be able to support parents and encourage them to foster their child's independence where it is apparent that a parent is showing extremes of protectiveness towards their child.

(ii) Parental neglect, indifference, low control and parental loss

As described in chapter 4, the research by Brown and Harris and their colleagues showed that prolonged lack of care in childhood was a causal factor in adult depression (Brown *et al.*, 1986b; Harris *et al.*, 1986). Following the loss of their mother by separation or death, those children who experienced either marked indifference or markedly low control from their fathers or substitute parents were three times more likely to be depressed when interviewed in adulthood than women with no such experiences (Brown *et al.*, 1986b). There was some indication, too, that the child who was showing signs of a helpless approach to life and one or more symptoms of childhood disturbance (truanting, bedwetting, stealing, fearfulness and so on) as well as experiencing a lack of care was especially likely to be depressed in adulthood (Harris *et al.*, 1987c). The assessment of parental indifference was based on the lack of parental interest shown in friends, school work, jobs and in adequate feeding and clothing of the child. Parental control, relating to restrictions and rules for behaviour, was judged to be low when supervision was so negligent that the child was left more or less to do as she pleased. This often occurred when the father alone had parental responsibility and was too busy or preoccupied to provide adequate care. It seemed that as mothers had usually hitherto had primary responsibility for child care, they were less likely than single fathers to neglect this function when trying to combine it with the role of breadwinner (Harris *et al.*, 1986).

From the point of view of prevention, this suggests that when a lack of care arises in the context of marital separation or parental death, some kind of support for the single parent may be particularly valuable. Support may help a bereaved parent to cope with his or her own feelings of loss, and thereby be better able to recognise their children's needs and vulnerability. Practical advice and assistance would also aid this process. The provision of a home help, information about financial benefits for single parents, advice and suggestions for managing the household, parental and financial tasks would be useful. Much of this support could be gained from voluntary befriending schemes, single parent advice groups and possibly the kinds of 'divorce workshops' that have gained a degree of popularity in American mental health centres.

However, as it was found to be the lack of care which followed the loss of a parent, rather than the loss itself, which explained the child's increased risk of depression in adulthood, the same vulnerability can be expected to result from lack of care in intact family homes (Harris *et al.*, 1986). And of course, most instances of lack of care will be in intact homes. These families are likely to be considerably more difficult to identify and to involve in preventive programmes. Mothers characterised by a high level of indifference towards their child or children are unlikely to look out for mother and toddler groups in their locality. It may be possible to reach some of this group if and when they attend health centres for antenatal care or child health check-ups. However, a more successful method may be through the health visitor, in her visits to mothers in their own homes. She is particularly well-placed to set up mothers' groups in her locality, and to encourage those she visits to attend. She could maximise the possibility that women would form supportive friendships which would outlast the group by bringing together women who seemed likely to get on well. And she could use these groups to provide some forms of education for parenthood. Alternatively, a more deliberate intervention in the form of a one-to-one (mother-to-mother) voluntary befriending scheme for mothers having marked parenting difficulties might be instituted. In fact several projects of this nature are currently operating and are having considerable success in improving the social, emotional and educational environment of the home (see chapter 9).

Some British health and social services are setting up family units, also specifically aimed at this hard-to-reach group. Staff will go to some trouble to enable families to attend. They aim to improve family relationships and parenting skills in order to reduce the possibility of family break-up. As yet their methods of doing so are ill-defined.

(iii) Substitute parenting

Between 1976 and 1980, there were over 95,000 children in the care of local authorities in England (DHSS, 1982). Roughly one-third of these children were in institutions (community homes and approved schools, or assessment centres), one-third boarded out with foster parents, and one-third in their own homes. Children who have been adopted after being received into care are not included in these figures. When the level of parenting available to a child is bad enough to make it appropriate for the state to intervene on his or her behalf, long-term planning to ensure continuing of good-quality substitute parenting should be essential. Adoption offers the most secure future. Otherwise, a long-term plan involving the natural parents and foster parents needs to be conceived with their cooperation as soon as possible (Rutter, 1982). Institutions cannot provide good parenting, but may be a valuable bridge between the child's own family and other permanent homes. The very high turnover of caregivers in institutional settings is perhaps the major way in which they differ from ordinary family life. Quinton and Rutter (1983) quote a figure of fifty or more parent figures during the first five years in a residential nursery as being common. They have made some suggestions for ways of improving the parenting provided, but there are serious practical problems in achieving a good standard of care.

Of course, these straightforward ideas mask substantial ethical and practical problems associated with state interference in family life. The complex issues which are raised cannot be satisfactorily considered within the brief discussions presented here. A detailed consideration of when and how it is in the child's best interests for the state to intervene in his family life can be found in Goldstein and colleagues (1973 and 1979). They expound their policy of minimal state interference to find the 'least detrimental available alternative' – one in which child placement and procedure for child placement 'maximises, in accord with the child's sense of time, the child's opportunity for being wanted and for maintaining on a continuous, unconditional and permanent basis, a relationship with at least one adult who is or will become the child's psychological parent' (Goldstein et al., 1979, p. 189). These far-reaching discussions recognise both the child's right to autonomous parents and family privacy, but also the parents' rights. They suggest that people other than the child's biological parents should be able to earn those rights if they have become the child's long-term caretakers.

If a good mothering experience can be provided even in late childhood, it can overturn all the bad experiences and provide a good model for the person's own mothering as well as boost her self-regard. Harris et al. (1987b) describes, by way of example, the case of a girl who had had numerous foster placements which broke down progressively more rapidly. The girl seemed likely to continue into adulthood with substantial social and emotional difficulties. However, when a particularly successful foster placement led to the girl's adoption the girl changed considerably. She thought more highly of herself and in later years was successful in establishing a mutually supportive and caring marital relationship. She was not judged as having an elevated risk of adult psychiatric disorder, despite her early disadvantage.

The transition period after leaving institutional care has also been documented as a critical time, when young people may be forced to return to the unhappy home situation from which they had been removed years earlier. Where this is the case, early marriage, often preceded by premarital pregnancy, is a common escape route for girls (Rutter *et al.*, 1983), and this in turn substantially raises the likelihood of adult depression (Harris *et al.*, 1987a). Practical support at the time at which young people raised in care are forced to leave their residential homes to help them settle into satisfactory new home environments, perhaps by helping them to get flats with friends or places in small half-way hostels with friends and supplying a realistic preparation for independent living, might avoid many difficulties. Additionally, a more flexible attitude by social services to enable the young person without fully satisfactory living arrangements to go to, to stay on as long as necessary at the home, would be preferable to sticking rigidly to a somewhat arbitrary age cut-off time. There may well be a case for social workers or child care workers to be appointed with this resettlement role as their particular brief.

According to Grosskurth (1984), some innovative schemes along these lines have already been set up by a few progressive British local authorities, but it seems that they are as yet rare, and reach only a minority of the people in need. She reports that while only a small proportion of all eighteen-year-olds live independently, a majority of those reared in care have to do so, and these are often ill-prepared, have meagre financial help and currently have limited prospects of finding work. Few authorities were felt to have a coherent policy on supporting their older children. Grosskurth suggests such a policy should include not only housing provision, but an adequate preparation for coping with independent living after years of dependent living in institutions. A disproportionate and disturbingly high number of care leavers join the ranks of the single homeless.

(iv) Premarital pregnancy, early marriage and 'planning'

There were at least 60,000 live births to teenage mothers in 1980 in England and Wales. A further 36,000 teenage pregnancies were aborted in the same year (Wells, 1983). Wells calculates that as approximately two-thirds of teenage pregnancies going to full term were reported to be unplanned in a study in South West England, effective contraception therefore has the potential for avoiding 76,000 unwanted teenage pregnancies each year.

Teenage mothers are more likely than older mothers to have an unstable family background, to have poor or no educational qualifi-cations, and to be unemployed at the time of conception (Wells, 1983). More successful education about birth control measures and more approachable advisory services may be part of the answer, but many unwanted pregnancies seem to occur among experienced contraceptors who give up without specifically wishing to become pregnant (Wells, 1983). An important factor in avoiding pre-marital pregnancy would seem to be the girl's own attitudes and behaviour in taking control of and planning her life. Quinton and Rutter's (1983) study of girls raised in care showed that girls who were 'planners' in other aspects of their lives were considerably less likely to become pregnant. Similarly, Harris and her colleagues (Brown *et al.*, 1986b; Harris *et al.*, 1987b) suggested that helpless attitudes and ways of thinking are a link between childhood lack of care, premarital pregnancy and depression. Quinton and Rutter (1983) have suggested that school experiences may be critical sources of self-esteem for children lacking supportive home lives, and that this in turn enhances their capacity to plan their lives.

An interesting, if somewhat methodologically weak, study by Flah-erty and his colleagues (1983) on adolescent pregnancies seems to be in line with this notion of planning ability. They compared groups of virgins, non-contraceptors, contraceptors and pregnant girls on their ability to anticipate the consequences of actions, to generate solutions and plan steps to implement them, in a variety of hypo-thetical problems unrelated to contraception. They found no group differences in the girls' abilities to anticipate consequences of actions. However, pregnant girls gave the least number of alternative solutions to the problems, and were least competent at describing the steps an imaginary protagonist should take to achieve her aims in five stories.

Together, these studies suggest that knowledge about contracep-tion and about family planning services, and the desire to become pregnant, by no means fully explain premarital pregnancy. In fact, Flaherty and his colleagues (1983) were unable to find any evidence that intervention programmes with teenage childbearers offering intensive family planning education had any success at all in preventing repeat pregnancies, though others have had less discouraging experiences (Osofsky *et al.*, 1973). Sex education in schools may therefore have most impact if it aims to discourage helpless attitudes, by emphasising to young people that they are in control of their own lives, encouraging them to see themselves as active rather than passive, and in discussing what they might do in the event of an unwanted pregnancy. This last issue is of course the last link in the chain leading to high vulnerability to depression. If the girl avoids becoming trapped, through an unwanted pregnancy, into an unsatisfactory lifestyle with an unsupportive or absent marital partner, she may still break out of the adverse chain of events.

(v) Interactive processes, problems of intervention

It seems clear that throughout the developmental period, certain factors can be identified which in certain circumstances will increase a person's future psychiatric risk. In nearly all instances, however, it is the chain of adverse circumstances with which the factor is associated which accumulate to generate this risk. Only if an intervention is effective not only in eliminating this factor, but also in transforming the person's lifestyle such that he or she is removed from this conveyor belt of risk, can the effects of the intervention be expected to be apparent ten or twenty years later. The difficulties in achieving such effective intervention can easily be imagined. This is not to say, however, that prevention is impossible, simply that preventive programmes need to concentrate not only on the removal or modification of isolated stresses, but also on the factors surrounding and responsible for such stresses, for these may be of equal or even greater importance in the development of later psychiatric disorders.

7
Approaches to prevention: supporting troubled persons

In spite of very real gains in knowledge, there is a long way to go before we can fully understand why one person is more likely to become mentally ill than another. Just how much is due to inherited characteristics, and how much to other biological factors or early childhood experiences is still uncertain. But personal characteristics are certainly not the whole story. Mental illness occurs in a context, and our understanding of factors in the current social environment which play a role in onset, recovery and relapse is growing. In particular, life events of certain kinds have been implicated in a wide range of disorder, and some of the evidence to establish their role has been described in earlier chapters. Environmental factors, as well as personal characteristics, affect the probability that events will be followed by disorder (and indeed also whether events will occur). And environmental factors provide an obvious focus for a consideration of preventive options. As is now possible with heart disease, perhaps preventive approaches will serve to increase the threshold for the appearance of illness. This chapter will consider personal resources for dealing with personal environmental challenges. The following chapter will extend the focus to consider the influence of factors in the wider social sphere – the effects of cultural values and practices.

Events, psychological distress and psychiatric disorder

Everyone experiences disturbing life events from time to time, and although they may cause a good deal of psychological distress, they cannot on the whole be considered to have a deleterious effect on health. In fact the reverse case can be argued. The person who creates a crisis in a relationship which is not going well such that the two part company and he or she is able to establish a more suitable and rewarding partnership may do much better than the person who avoids crises and settles for a far from ideal partner. The person who, despite their concern about the loss of a company pension, leaves an organisation after many years of service in a disliked job to try a new field may well do better, in health terms, than the person who sticks it out in the miserable job. Even apparently adverse and uncontrollable events like suddenly needing to undergo urgent major surgery may well be an essentially positive experience if dealt with well. Once it becomes clear that recovery is likely, it may, for instance, lead a person to re-examine their lifestyle and come to positive decisions about how they would like to improve it and make more of its good features.

It makes no sense to contemplate a general policy of reducing adverse events in people's lives, even if it were possible, unless perhaps they were crises which might unavoidably lead to the person becoming trapped into a highly stressful lifestyle. Perhaps, for instance, a case could be made for discouraging risks that might lead to a person's loss of employment, if their chances of gaining another job were remote. Similarly, for the teenage girl from a strongly Catholic family it might be particularly important that she avoid pregnancy in a relationship with a boy to whom she felt sure she would not like to be married. Such events would be likely to result in long-term adversity – unemployment and financial hardship for the first person, loss of family support at the same time as facing the prospects of single parenthood or marrying an unsuitable man 'for the sake of the baby' for the second. Being trapped by such circumstances may well increase the individual's likelihood of suffering a psychiatric disorder, because, by definition, they would become unable or restricted in capacity to deal with the developing difficulties.

However, earlier chapters have shown that life events are implicated in a range of psychiatric disorder, and that to a certain extent it is possible to specify the broad type of event which will precede a particular type of disorder. Events which have been linked with depression, for instance, are those which, in the context of the person's current life, seem to pose a marked degree of long-term threat following a loss or disappointment, not least in the sense of failure to restore or replace that which has been lost. The threat may be loss or disappointment concerning a cherished idea or aspiration, object, person or role. Very often, they are events which are perceived as moving the individual to the periphery of a social group, in effect into a more emotionally or socially isolated position (Gilbert, 1984). Events which are severely threatful only for a few days, or which are of a relatively mild or even positive nature, are unlikely to be associated with depression (see chapter 4).

Many threatening events arise from social disadvantage (financial, housing, employment). Many others might be described as acts of God – receiving a diagnosis of multiple sclerosis, for example. Leaving to one side the possibility of major political and economic changes, most events of the sort implicated in depression are probably not amenable to prevention at an individual level.

Events which have been implicated in schizophrenia are of a more everyday nature (although it is possible that many also have a private meaning), and a very wide range of emotionally arousing events may trigger a relapse. The event might not have any obvious long-term adverse significance and may in fact have seemingly positive rather than negative features, such as the reappearance and request to renew contact with a lover with whom a person had had an intense relationship a few years earlier. How can such events be prevented? Furthermore, where either depression or schizophrenia are provoked or triggered by an event, disorder typically follows so rapidly that intervention after the event and before the emergence of disorder is unlikely to be a practical possibility. If it took a couple of weeks to trace and arrange to visit all the closest relatives of the victims of a train disaster, say, those most likely to become severely depressed might already have done so. In which case, intervention must aim to help troubled people, as the title of this chapter suggests, so that their depression does not become seriously prolonged and severe beyond their 'normal' experience of grief.

However, although it seems at first sight that prospects for prevention associated with life events are bleak, there are nevertheless a number of realistic possibilities, and it is important to go through these. To begin with, people who have suffered from schizophrenia are readily identifiable, and it may well at times be possible to make the lives of this high-risk group less eventful. For instance, if good supportive accommodation and a job with a sympathetic employer could be found, this would immediately reduce the potential range of home and work-related events. Moreover, it might be possible to resolve some of the difficulties that might arise before, say, eviction or redundancy became real possibilities.

Many, if not most, events implicated in depression do not occur out of the blue. While this may not mean they are preventable, there is at least the possibility of fortifying the individual against their effects. And certain existing circumstances often appear to influence the likelihood of their occurrence. Previous difficulty in maintaining a pregnancy through to a live birth will be likely to be associated with a greater risk of a third or fourth miscarriage than if the woman's previous pregnancies had been trouble-free. Hence some kind of additional support, information or psychological preparation for further failure might be instituted, and this might be valuable in preventive terms. Marital break-up is often, if not usually, preceded by some years of turbulence and unreliability on the part of one or both partners. A person whose poor health has caused progressively longer and more frequent absences from work will increasingly be at risk of losing his or her job. Such circumstances might be called 'event-producing situations'. Furthermore, a history of failure in an important aspect of one's life will also be likely to affect the meaning and interpretation put on further failures, and increases the likelihood that in the context of the person's life, the event *will* pose a marked and long-term threat of loss – in the first example above, of the possibility of becoming a parent.

In fact, it is increasingly clear that in formulating realistic possibilities for prevention around life events in the person's current life, it will be essential to consider the person's past history. It is the long-term lead-up to events which is often critical. The identification of certain antecedent risk factors is needed in order that a high-risk group can be selected for whom events of certain types may indeed provoke or precipitate psychiatric disorder. Such factors may include, for instance, a previous experience of loss which was dealt with badly, unresolved grief, past experience of failure, a lack of a sense of self-efficacy, a low self-esteem, a previous history of psychiatric disorder, and an absence of close relationships established over a long period of time. The identification of risk and the reasons for high risk may then point the way towards meaningful and constructive attempts to intervene.

One important feature of such factors is that they will tend to shape the person's capacity to cope with adverse circumstances. That is, to take actions to resolve difficulties and to draw on psychological resources to control the meaning of the event and to control the distress with which it is associated (Pearlin and Schooler, 1978).

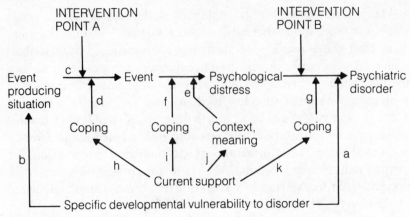

Figure 7.1

Research on crisis support invariably focuses on the notion of coping, but the complexity of this idea is not always reflected in intervention studies. Coping behaviour is associated with current external resources (money, information, practical help), which also relate to available supportive relationships, and with internal psychological resources (confidence, experience, knowledge).

Essentially three sets of concepts can be brought together in relation to life events to help conceptualise possibilities for prevention. Certain *qualities* of events have been linked to a raised probability that a particular psychiatric disorder will develop shortly afterwards. Certain *circumstances* are particularly likely to lead to the occurrence of such events. Certain individual psychosocial characteristics will affect the *interpretation* of and response to a given event. It might be argued, therefore, that if sufficient was known about people's lives, it would be possible to allocate the population to one of four risk groups:

(1) those who have recently experienced an event to which they were particularly vulnerable;

(2) those whose circumstances make them highly likely to experience an event to which they are particularly vulnerable;

(3) those who are vulnerable to particular types of event, but whose circumstances either make their occurrence unlikely, or provide resources for dealing with the event should it occur;

(4) those who are not especially vulnerable to any specific kind of stress.

The first two groups are those for whom preventive intervention may turn out to be justified. Figure 7.1 illustrates in a general way

the likely sequence of contributing factors, and the two most promising points of intervention.

It is not put forward as a definitive model for how coping, support
and events interrelate in the genesis of psychiatric disorder, because
the issues are so complex that the diagram could be redrawn in
several different ways and indicate several other likely relationships.
Rather, its purpose is to simplify the issues sufficiently to be able to
put a coherent structure on the following discussions about some of
the ways in which the various factors interrelate, and the possibility
of intervention. The subheadings throughout this chapter focus on
each of the factors (a–k) in Figure 7.1 in turn, and their effects on
the likelihood that events will be followed by illness.

Specific developmental vulnerability to disorder

The concept of a specific vulnerability is commonly used to explain
why person A who experiences a severe event becomes depressed,
but persons B, C, D and E do not. Or why person D, who experiences
a relatively minor but intrusive event which would have no adverse
consequences for persons A, B, C and E, becomes floridly psychotic
(arrow a, Figure 7.1). Possible explanations include a biological
predisposition to a specific disorder; the particular threat embodied
in the event to the person's long-term plans and purposes; the
significance of the event in the context of the person's previous
history of failure or loss; and personal characteristics like a lack of
confidence or self-esteem. In schizophrenia, the first of these is the
one we know most about. In depression, less is known about
biological vulnerability, but knowledge is accumulating about other
explanations (see chapters 4 and 5).

Event-producing situations

Some specific developmental vulnerability factors are partly explain-
able in terms of their effects on the lifestyle of the individual, and
on the extent to which the person is likely to experience threatening
life events (arrow b, Figure 7.1). A helpless approach to life and a
low sense of self-esteem are two factors which have been suggested
as being associated with a raised risk of depression following threatening life events (see chapter 4). These same factors might also make
it more likely that a person *will* experience the sorts of events to

which they will be vulnerable. One of the explanations put forward by Brown *et al.* (1986b) for the link between childhood lack of care, premarital pregnancy and adult risk of depression, for instance, was that the early adversities militated against the child developing a sense of control over her life, and exercising it. Hence unwanted pregnancy was more likely to occur, the girl was also unlikely to deal positively with this event, and likely to drift into an unsuitable, unsupportive marital relationship or single parenthood, and experience adverse events linked to her unsatisfactory lifestyle. In this event-producing situation the risk of depression was considerably increased.

Other event-producing situations are unrelated to an individual's approach to life or personality characteristics. Old age, for instance, is a time characterised by frequent losses of one's peers, a loss of function and independence, health problems and, not infrequently, increasing financial hardship. Many ongoing difficult social circumstances, whether or not a direct result of the person's approach to life, may also erupt at some point into major crises. A large family in unsuitable housing with financial hardship is more likely than families with greater material resources to find certain events stressful, such as unexpected financial crises leading to debt. Such families are also more likely to have dangerous forms of heating, and less likely to be insured against damage by fire. Poverty is clearly an event-producing situation. Working in an industry that is in decline in an area where alternative employment is scarce makes job loss and consequent financial difficulty increasingly probable. Caring for a relative with a progressive, relapsing illness or terminal condition makes future related adverse events almost certain (arrow c, Figure 7.1).

It is undoubtedly possible to identify many event-producing situations. The health services will know of people treated for psychiatric illnesses and a follow-up service or routine visit from community nurses should be able to recognise obviously unsatisfactory living circumstances. Social services often know families in extreme financial difficulty. Employers could provide advance warning of intended plant closures or major reorganisation. Hospital staff will have some of their major surgery planned many weeks in advance. They will know of patients likely to die in the near future and of patients recently permanently handicapped by their illness or injury. Old people's homes will know of plans to move elderly people from their own or relatives' homes into local authority or private care. Police will know families of men arrested for criminal offences. Gas and electricity accounts departments will know those customers whose financial difficulties are going to lead them to a cessation of supply. Of course, serious issues of confidentiality would have to be resolved, but the potential for recognition is clearly there.

However, as has already been made clear, preventive programmes cannot be planned for everyone likely to face such events. Additional knowledge is required to specify more closely the smaller proportion of troubled people who would be most susceptible to developing psychiatric disorder in the context of particular events.

Coping in event-producing situations

The aim of coping responses in event-producing situations (arrow d, Figure 7.1) must be either to reduce the likelihood that a severe event will occur (perhaps by seeking marriage guidance counselling to help resolve marital difficulties), or to prepare oneself emotionally for the distressing event which is likely or certain to occur (compulsory redundancy, say). But unfortunately there are few descriptive accounts of people's efforts to reduce the likelihood that an event will occur, perhaps because effective responses are self-evident, or because they are not easily assessed by investigators in that successful action will have removed the difficulty. Pearlin and his colleagues have discussed the effectiveness of commonly used coping responses to various chronic role strains of the sort likely to erupt at any time into major events (Pearlin and Schooler, 1978; Pearlin et al., 1981). During interviews with more than 2,000 adults in Chicago they attempted to identify the conflicts, frustrations and other role strains encountered by parents, married couples, workers and breadwinners, the coping behaviours used to attempt to minimise their impact, and any current symptoms of depression and anxiety. It might have been expected that strategies aimed to change the stressful circumstances themselves would be an important feature of the coping responses they uncovered. In fact, very few responses of this kind were identified. It seems unlikely, however, that this is a true reflection of the significance of such behaviour. But leaving this to one side, Pearlin and Schooler do deal with some methods of mentally restructuring the meaning of the difficulty that are commonly used to reduce distress. These strategies were exemplified in statements on the part of respondents such as 'count your blessings', or 'we're all in the same boat', and in methods such as perceiving hardship as the forerunner of an easier future, or devaluing the importance of aspects which are noxious (such as an unpleasant boss and colleagues) and magnifying good aspects (such as the convenient location and reasonable pay of the job).

These are all examples of ways in which people learn to live with long-term social difficulties which they have not been able to change. Many specific events also have something of this quality, such as requiring major surgery or needing to sell up and move from one's home to cover a business loss. Because such potentially distressing events are predictable, but unavoidable, they are an ideal focus for an investigation of coping behaviours. The way the time leading up to the event is used, and the success of the coping behaviours employed, may considerably affect its impact (Parkes, 1982a). Indeed, the exercise of such anticipatory coping was one of Caplan's central notions for primary prevention. The specialist draws the person's attention to the details of an impending hazard

> and attempts to evoke ahead of time a vivid anticipation of the experience with its associated feelings of anxiety, tension, depression and deprivation. He then helps them to begin to envisage possible ways of reacting, including mastery of negative feelings. When the experience itself arrives, the hazards will be attenuated because they have been made familiar by being anticipated, and the individuals will already have been set on the path of healthy coping responses. (Caplan, 1964, p. 84)

Of course, it is not always helpful to prepare for the worst if there is a possibility that the event may not occur. The good general does not admit the possibility of defeat, and a doctor would rarely advise a patient that his tumour is probably cancerous until the possibility that it is benign has been ruled out. However, as Parkes (1982a) points out, morale-boosting optimism is sometimes taken to absurd lengths, and much of the undoubted success of the hospice approach to the care of terminally ill patients stems from the recognition of this fact. Here, staff appreciate that both fear and grief in the patient and his relatives can be reduced through anticipating the fact that they do not have much longer together and that this time can be used constructively to work through some of their anxieties and other distressing emotions. This can be contrasted with hospital care where either the patient or his relatives or both are not informed about the imminence of his death. The possible consequence of such ignorance has been described by Parkes and Weiss (1983) in terms of the 'unanticipated death syndrome'. They characterise this as a combination of shock, anger and persisting illusions of the continuing presence of the dead person. Cameron and Parkes (1983) cite, by way of example, the death of a woman who had spent her last weekend at home with her husband discussing plans for the future while sitting in the sun to regain her strength. Her husband had not realised that she was dying, and the subsequent shock was so great that he became unable to care for his six-year-old daughter who also began to lose weight and perform badly at school. Preoccupied with fears and thoughts of his wife, he was distressed, angry and suicidally inclined.

But how does a person normally prepare himself for frightening and distressing events? Some important insights have been gained from the study of people who voluntarily undertake frightening events as part of a sport.

Epstein (1983) used the sport of parachute jumping as a natural laboratory for the study of fear and its mastery. Because the event (the jump) is known in advance, the effects of practice and mastery could be assessed, and efforts made to influence the coping process. The fear of novice and experienced parachutists was measured at several stages prior to a jump, using both the subject's own ratings of fear, and GSR scores (galvanic skin response, or the electrical resistance of the skin which is a physiological indication of emotional tension). For novices, anxiety tended to mount steadily from the day before a jump to the moment of jumping. However, for experienced parachutists, anxiety was usually high on the day before the jump but then steadily reduced to a low level by the time of the jump. However, if a number of unexpected new experiences and distractions were introduced in this intervening period, the anxiety of experienced parachutists returned to the novice pattern. Epstein concluded that management of stress among the experienced parachutists was not due to their repeated exposure to jumping in the manner of a conditioned response, but was a consequence of an active coping process that on each occasion was used to prepare them for the coming jump.

He goes on to argue that we can learn to cope with the anxiety associated with an anticipated event or with a recent unanticipated event by mastering progressively greater amounts of stress. It is possible to attend to moderately stressful cues and mentally explore and master their threat before proceeding to attend to more salient stimuli. Those failing to take themselves through such graded stress inoculation may be reduced to falling back on an all-or-none defence mechanism in which awareness of the stressful event is completely blocked out, or is experienced in overwhelming intensity. He suggests that this maladaptive strategy helps to explain the traumatic neuroses which sometimes follow events like bereavement, and which can be contrasted with successful adjustment in which the individual works through grief triggered by indirect reminders and gradually progresses to being able to respond to stronger reminders of the deceased. Novice parachutists who blocked out fear completely up to the moment of the jump were often overcome with an overwhelming and incapacitating anxiety such that they not only did not jump but decided to give up jumping forever.

Such stress inoculation in the form of graded exposure to increasing levels of stress is believed by Epstein to be a natural healing process of the mind. But it is also a procedure which can be taught. It is already widely used in teaching people to overcome a range of fears, from phobias, dating anxiety, and anxiety prior to undergoing surgery, to readjusting to normal living habits for victims of rape (see Meichenbaum and Jaremko, 1983).

Context and meaning

For the professional footballer whose plans and aspirations require physical fitness, an accident involving a permanent disability is likely to be seen as disastrous. For an office worker uninterested in sport the implications may well be less profound. It would not be surprising if the loss of a job for a middle-aged manager who would have difficulty finding other similar employment within his field of expertise and at his age and occupational level was experienced as highly distressing. To a younger worker who had not yet specialised and could more easily be re-employed without seriously losing status, the threat might be less serious. As a woman's teenage children leave home, she may interpret the loss of the first as a welcome freedom. When the last child leaves and she no longer has any daily parenting responsibilities, she may experience a crisis over the loss of status as mother, particularly if she has no other clearly defined role.

These examples illustrate, albeit crudely, the way the meanings of events (see arrow e, Figure 7.1) tend to link to a person's plans, purposes and roles to which they are more or less committed. But while the perceived effect of events on future plans may be a critical factor in the development of affective disorder, such general interpretations of events do not appear to offer much scope for intervention. As already noted, events on the whole cannot be prevented, and it will often be extremely difficult to recognise those for whom they present a particular threat to future aspirations. The middle-aged manager might have well-thought-out ideas about how he would spend his enforced early retirement. Likewise the middle-aged mother may also have had aspirations which had for many years been put aside until her parenting responsibilities were at an end.

However, events may also pose a particular threat when their interpretation is coloured by the past, rather than the future. And here the implications for prevention become somewhat more realistic. For instance, there is evidence that a long history of failure in an important area of a person's life makes them particularly vulnerable to depression in the context of a major loss or disappointment which could be interpreted as further evidence of their lack of competence. In their prospective study of 400 working-class women with children in North London, Brown and his colleagues (1987) found a threefold increased risk of depression to follow severe events which arose from a long-standing social difficulty compared to women experiencing the same kind of event but without such a prior history. A long experience of management problems with a child, for instance, increased the chance that a crisis such as the child's arrest for a criminal offence would provoke an episode of depression in the mother.

Silver and Wortman's review of research (1980) on how people adjust to major losses suggests something similar. Past experience of losses of the same nature as a current loss was found to reduce the person's capacity to deal with the current loss. Yet it is often argued that the successful adjustment to a major loss makes the person *better* able to deal with future losses (e.g. Caplan, 1964). Their findings therefore seemed puzzling and they looked for possible explanations. They suggested that the repeated occurrence of similar losses might increase the likelihood of believing oneself to blame for the event. Perhaps the rationalisation the person devises for coping with the first loss is shattered by the second loss. Perhaps the person experiences an overwhelming sense of injustice which renders them less capable of dealing with the problem a second time. This connection between past experience relevant to the current event and the interpretation of the event has also been described in studies of grief following bereavement. Parkes and Weiss (1983) described the contexts in which clinical depression was particularly likely to follow bereavement. Circumstances which may lead to chronic grief or clinging, for instance, included a previous ambivalent relationship with the deceased or a previous relationship in which the survivor felt either inferior or insecure.

As many as half the severe events documented by Brown and Harris in their studies of women in inner-city areas arose from long-standing difficulties. This suggests that it may sometimes be possible to identify people likely to experience events which will match a long-standing difficulty before the occurrence of the event itself: a pregnant woman, for instance, who has previously had three miscarriages.

Coping with the event and the distress

Once an event with marked long-term threat has occurred, there are two stages of coping. Firstly, the event itself must be dealt with (arrow f, Figure 7.1), and secondly, irrespective of its threatening implications, there will be coping responses for getting through and managing the resulting distress (arrow g, Figure 7.1). At both stages, coping can have behavioural and psychological aspects. The behavioural aspect is obvious. Faced with worrying medical symptoms in one's child, signs that an elderly parent can no longer cope alone in their own home, or the sight of flames consuming the house around you – what you *do* is crucial! And the success of actions in these circumstances would serve to reduce the potential long-term threat associated with the event. The person who stays calm and takes steps to control the fire, or manages to get their child to the hospital before their appendix bursts, will undoubtedly be reducing the chances that the event will have serious long-term implications. On the other hand, the person who discovers a lump under their skin but is too frightened to go to the doctor lest he diagnose cancer will be perpetuating the threatening situation – and this would hold even if the lump was in fact benign.

However, should the house burn to the ground and the lump finally be diagnosed as malignant cancer, the role for behavioural coping strategies is clearly reduced. There may still be some possibilities, however, perhaps by filling as much of the waking day as possible with exhausting and demanding activity to reduce the time which can be given to introspection.

There is a considerable literature on the psychological strategies that can be effective in dealing with crises. Pearlin and his colleagues (1981) found that the same sorts of cognitive strategies which were commonly successfully employed by people adapting to chronic role strains were also effective in helping to neutralise the threat of severe events. About half their original sample had been given a second interview four years after the first. During the interval, eighty-eight had been made redundant, downgraded or fired from work. A statistical procedure, step-by-step regression analysis, correlated particular coping behaviours reported to have been used in response to this event and ten symptoms of depression assessed at the second interview. They concluded that two kinds of response serving to control the meaning of the event by neutralising its economic threat were helpful. The first involved the person comparing his lot with those in a worse economic position, or with times in the past in his own life when circumstances had been worse, or in the future when they might be worse. Where they reported that they were able to see the present as better, existing symptoms were lower than average. A second strategy involved demeaning the importance of money and monetary success. Both approaches therefore involved attributing a new meaning to the situation. Leaving aside the problem of time order in the research, and whether their findings do indeed reveal genuine causal effects of coping behaviour, it is unclear how relevant such strategies would be for the general run of threatening events. It is less easy to see, for instance, how the meaning of a loss such as bereavement could be so readily reinterpreted, or whether such attempts do much to reduce the risk of depression.

There is in fact little evidence that coping responses play a role in the aetiology of major psychiatric disorder since it has not been possible so far to conduct experiments. Investigators are therefore forced to reconstruct complex behavioural and psychological processes after the event has occurred and sometimes after the disorder itself. It is always possible, therefore, that too much weight has been given to the reported cognitive responses. However, research concerning bereavement has been particularly revealing because some prospective work *is* possible.

Terminally ill people are not only identifiable, but their closest relatives are also easily located in hospital and hospice settings and from their contacts with clergymen and general practitioners. Two components of necessary grief work have been identified, and have been summarised by Parkes (1982b). Firstly, the bereaved person needs to accept, express and work through his feelings of sorrow and hostility, and to review his relationship with the deceased. Secondly, he must extricate himself from his involvement with the deceased and search out new relationships as sources of rewarding interaction.

Silver and Wortman (1980), in their review of research on how people cope with a range of such major losses, conclude that two resources in particular seem to have some generalisable benefit. The opportunity to talk about feelings and experiences, and to ventilate anxieties, sadness, anger or despair is important, as is the ability to find some personal meaning in the experience – for instance, following the death of one's child, believing that his or her suffering and treatment may in some way help other children with the same affliction in the future. In general, research suggests that in the immediate wake of unexpected news of a major loss, such as finding oneself permanently disabled after a car accident, denial may also, in the short term, be an adaptive response as a means of buying time for the individual (Adams and Lindemann, 1974).

Conclusions about coping responses which have a protective effect against a wide range of events are more easily obtained when the events are likely to be associated with acute anxiety and fear rather than depression (e.g. Jaremko, 1983). Jaremko notes that the person's first response to the threat will usually be a physiological one – the pounding heart, as the body prepares for fight or flight. This leads to an automatic psychological appraisal of the situation as threatening, and in turn to frightening thoughts and images, which in their turn feed back to maintain a rapid heart rate. Physical skills such as slow breathing or chewing gum can reduce the heart rate and thereby lessen the automatic appraisal of the stressor as threatening. The person may then use psychological strategies such as a sequence of self-statements to change the way he perceives the stressor and ensure that thoughts and images are less anxiety-provoking (Jaremko, 1983). This active search for alternatives may include attempts to convert the threat into a challenge that promises growth and achievement (Lazarus, 1976). Finally he can use 'cognitive restructuring' to replace negative self-statements like 'It's going to be awful' with positive statements like 'I'm sure I'll manage' (Jaremko, 1983).

These cognitive coping strategies might be viewed as internal resources for dealing with threatening events and chronic social difficulties. As such they can be separated from external resources such as practical help, information and emotional support.

Social support

The extensive literature on the complex issue of social support has been reviewed many times. That social support may play a major role in modifying the deleterious effects of stress on health and may also influence other aspects of health behaviour such as use of health services and the following of medical advice appears now to be widely accepted. It is common for reviewers to cite evidence of effects on physical pathology from a study by Cassel (1976) who reported an increased prevalence of hypertension and stroke in groups deficient in social supports, and from work by Berkman and Syme (1979) who reported a raised mortality among adults deficient in social ties in a sample of 6,928 individuals studied prospectively over a nine-year period. Investigators focusing on the ill-effects of life stress on mental health have also demonstrated the protective effects of social support (for example Cobb, 1976; Brown and Harris, 1978). Gore (1978), and Bolton and Oatley (1987) have shown how various kinds of social support can cushion the impact of unemployment. Others have shown its protective influence for the bereaved (Raphael, 1977) and against chronic work stress (House, 1981).

However, the research findings have not always been consistent and there has been controversy over their significance. A number of investigators have failed to find the expected correlations between lack of support, stress and psychiatric disorder shown in Figure 7.1. Some careful reviews of the evidence have helped to clarify the position. By taking into account the adequacy of the research designs, ruling out findings from small samples, weak measures and poor statistical analysis, Kessler and McLeod (1984) revealed a considerable amount of agreement about the positive effects of support. From a review of twenty-five normal population surveys, they conclude that emotional support and perceived availability of support are both likely to buffer the effects of stress on health. But in the absence of high stress they find no reason to conclude that emotional support has any general influence on mental health.

Kessler and McLeod also found plausible evidence in three studies that the buffering effects of emotional support might be at least as important in circumstances of chronic strain as for people facing the acute stress of major events. Furthermore, they suggest that some researchers who have reported correlations between emotional support and health in the absence of life events might in fact be picking up a correlation between chronic strain and support.

Eight of the studies reviewed by Kessler and McLeod considered the effects of support on stress provided by affiliative networks as opposed to that from intimate relationships, that is, by assessing number of friends, community involvement and social activities. They found no pervasive effect of membership in affiliative networks in the presence of stress. They concluded, however, that it was possible that social networks have a modest association with mental health even though they offer little protection against acute stress. This would concur with the conclusions of reviews of the much larger literature on support and health which does not specifically consider the effects of stress. It may also be that informal support networks are valuable in managing chronic strain. For instance, Neighbors and his colleagues (1983) found that prayer and the church were the most commonly cited responses of black Americans facing marked economic and family difficulties.

While evidence that social support in some way short-circuits the illness response to stress is now considerable, the nature of the support and the way in which it provides its effect remain matters for dispute. Whether its effect is direct or indirect, as an antecedent or buffer, or whether it is availability or perceived availability that is important, are all issues which have been controversial.

(i) What quality of a relationship is protective?

House (1981) describes three ways in which social ties can be supportive. They can provide: functional support (tangible help such as money, services); informational support (advice, knowledge); and emotional support. Gottlieb (1983) describes the latter as 'an expression of reliable alliance with the respondents and a genuine concern for their well-being'. But while some obviously see social support as something easily recognisable, emphasising that the supporter must actually be present or accessible during stressful episodes (e.g. Cassel, 1976), others, like Cobb, conceive of support in less down-to-earth terms. Cobb argues that social support arises in the eye of the beholder, and is anything that influences the person to perceive himself as the recipient of positive affect; any information 'leading the subject to believe that he is cared for and loved . . . esteemed and valued . . .' (Cobb, 1976, p. 300).

Robert Weiss, who has conducted a number of intensive studies of adult relationships, has set out to identify the provisions of different kinds of social ties. Close, intimate relationships such as may exist between marriage partners, are contrasted with those with other family members, friends and wider social contacts. By way of illustration, he described the loneliness experienced by many recently separated couples, even when they have longed for the divorce, and despite a great deal of support from companions. Another observation was of the isolation which can be experienced by the housewife, despite a close and happy marriage, when a move of residence deprives her of the company of friends. Both intimate and friendship ties are therefore considered potentially important for well-being. Two other types of bond are relationships organised around investments in the welfare of another (ordinarily one's own children); and relationships organised around an acceptance of someone as a valid source of support and guidance – the boss at work, the general practitioner perhaps, or the vicar (Weiss, 1982).

Weiss believes friendships to be important in so far as they reflect attitudes and behaviour that are supportive of the individual's own beliefs, and they provide a reassurance of self-worth by virtue of their acceptance. Close attachments foster feelings of comfort and security, while investments in the well-being of others provides a rationale for one's continued striving, a sense of continuity through time, and an opportunity for reliving and mastering unsatisfactory early experiences of one's own. He argues, therefore, that social ties may differ radically in function and should not be considered to provide some unitary benefit in terms of concepts such as emotional support. He also emphasises the need to take into account the costs of relationships, and the possibility that in some instances, apparently supportive relationships can have a negative impact on well-being.

Research on the development of various types of psychiatric disorder has so far suggested that close relationships tend to play the most crucial role in increasing or decreasing vulnerability. In the context of the earlier discussion on meaning, this might be interpreted as those relationships which help to establish and sustain a person's self-esteem in areas to which he is highly committed. But it appears that it is more often the negative effect of a close relationship, rather than any positive effect, that is of significance in determining psychiatric risk. Firstly, as the research on the course of schizophrenia described in chapter 5 showed, a high level of criticism and overinvolvement expressed by the key close relative in the home increased the likelihood that a person who had previously been treated for schizophrenia would suffer an acute relapse of florid symptoms. Low expressed emotion, on the other hand, and a positive approach to fostering social competence by relatives could, along with maintenance neuroleptic medication, reduce vulnerability to relapse to a low level (Leff et al., 1982; Falloon et al., 1982). Secondly, not only have Brown and his colleagues (1986a) confirmed that it is a close relationship that plays the key protective role in the development of depression (regular contact, fair level of confiding), but they also found that it was essential to consider both positive and negative aspects of such relationships for any satisfactory understanding. For instance, women with a marital relationship characterised by negative interaction (discord, tension, coldness and indifference) were found to be over three times more likely to become depressed after a severe event (35 per cent versus 10 per cent) than married women with a better relationship (Brown et al., 1986a). Thirdly, discordant marital relationships have been linked with a raised rate of psychiatric problems in the children (Rutter, 1981). And finally, a lack of interest in and control over their children on the part of parents has been argued to be a vulnerability factor for these children in adult depression (see chapter 4). It therefore seems that not only is the absence of close supportive others linked to vulnerability, but so too can be the presence of close unsupportive others.

However, there are further complexities as described in a recent paper by Brown and his colleagues (1986a) who explain why even the presence of seemingly good close relationships sometimes fails to be protective against depression. They show how important it is to consider the objectively quantifiable support provided within a relationship during a crisis. In their longitudinal study, they were surprised how many of the women who had been considered to have a supportive marital relationship when first interviewed became depressed after a later crisis. When the lives of the women were examined in more detail, this finding was explained; quite often, support at the time of their first contact with the woman was not translated into effective support in a crisis in the follow-up year. Married women were more likely than single mothers to be let down in this way, and such women were particularly likely to develop depression. Indeed, the high risk of depression among women let down by a husband was not mitigated by any other form of support.

Married women whose husbands provided the support expected of them, however, had a low risk of depression following life events. And for women in other circumstances, there was evidence that other types of support could be protective too. Married women who had not been receiving support from their husband when they were first interviewed, and were therefore not expecting support from him during subsequent crises, had a much reduced risk of depression if they received help from someone else whom they had named as very close at the first interview. Single mothers who had named a 'true' very close friend were also less likely to become depressed than single mothers without such friendships. Other research findings also suggest that less intimate ties can, under certain circumstances, be important. For instance, bereaved adults experience higher than expected levels of illness in the year following the death of their spouse, and among those most at risk of lasting psychiatric problems are people without a network of friends or relatives to whom they may turn for consolation (Parkes and Brown, 1972). Parkes's (1980) review of random allocation bereavement counselling studies indicated that guidance offered to such socially isolated individuals by trained professionals (or volunteers backed by professionals) could reduce their psychiatric risk (see chapter 9).

In general, the research is clear in showing the critical role of support in the development of depression, but that the relationship between support, crises and depression is far more complex than many researchers have previously conveyed.

*(ii) At what stage in the development of adverse events and psychological
distress is social support most important?*

The possibility of mounting preventive interventions to reduce
psychiatric risk will depend on information about the timing, as well
as the quality of effective support. Is the existence of a supportive
relationship before an event the critical factor, or can new supportive
relationships mobilised at the time of the event be effective? Perhaps
both are important in different ways. Existing ties may help to reduce
the number of events experienced (arrow h, Figure 7.1), reduce the
likelihood that events will be perceived as stressful (arrow j), and
provide emotional support after the event (arrows i and k). But mutual
aid organisations which have proliferated over recent decades are
based on an assumption that practical and highly specific emotional
support after the event, and from new social relationships, is helpful.

Research which has attempted to untangle these issues has not,
by and large, employed sufficiently sophisticated methods to clarify
the picture. Two often-cited studies are illustrative of the problems
of measuring support and assessing its timing, and therefore the
mechanisms through which it exerts its effects. Gore (1978) studied
the impact of unemployment at five points in time leading up to and
following the shutdown of two companies. Six weeks before and
immediately after the closedown was assumed to be a more stressful
time for the 100 men than one and two years later when 90 per
cent of them had found alternative employment. Social support was
assessed from a thirteen-item index covering the individual's perception of wife, friends and relatives as supportive or unsupportive,
frequency of activity with them, and perceived opportunity to talk
about problems and engage in satisfying social activities. Depression,
self-blame, number of pre-defined illness symptoms, and level of
serum cholesterol were also assessed.

One of the two companies was sited in a rural community, the
other in an urban environment. Men in the rural setting had longer
periods of unemployment, but fewer symptoms of depression,
suggesting that the broad social context played a role in adaptation
(Gore, 1978, p. 159). The rural men were found to have a higher
average rating of social support, and to live in a more cohesive
community judged by an atmosphere of concern about the threat to
its economic base which was not apparent in the urban area.
However, despite a wealth of fascinating data, she was unable to

untangle the causal sequence and be sure about what came first in order to conclude when and how support had been protective.

Lin and his colleagues (1979) also set out to explain why support might be protective among 121 men and 49 women randomly selected from a Chinese-American community in the USA. They assessed life events using the Holmes and Rahe checklist which ranks events according to the life change involved rather than their negative implications, and therefore includes seemingly positive events such as marriage. Their concept of support was also very broad, and their assessment more of a quantitive than a qualitive one. It included, for example, frequency of talking to neighbours, involvement in 'Chinese activities', and number of close friends living nearby. High support was found to be associated with a low rate of illness, and a high level of events with a high rate of illness. They argue that support acted as an antecedent protective factor, but as their data was not longitudinal, the relationships they found are open to alternative explanations.

As described earlier, Brown and his colleagues (1986a) have argued that they now have good evidence that the prior existence of a close supportive relationship is protective against depression if that person provides the support expected of them at the time of a crisis. Although the crucial relationships were pre-existing, and of a close, confiding quality, their protective effect derived from the support during the crisis. This means that it cannot be ruled out that new supportive relationships established at the time of a crisis might also sometimes be beneficial. It may be that only when key supportive figures are lacking, or have been lost, that others in the wider social network (the health visitor, 'befriender' or social worker) can have a protective effect.

The importance of support is almost certainly to some extent bound up with self-esteem and the ability of the individual to cope with difficulties as they arise (Brown *et al.*, 1986a; Pearlin *et al.*, 1981) Given that adverse life events can bring about affective disorders, this is hardly surprising as a general conclusion. However, the reverse situation seems equally, if not more important, and unsupportive, discordant close relationships can contribute to a negative self-esteem.

There is still a great deal to be learned about support, and there is no doubt that personal characteristics are also important. Much controversy surrounds the relative importance of internal factors (such as personality, intelligence and knowledge), and external factors (like social support) in determining coping skills. The research by Henderson in Australia, described in chapter 4, has provoked considerable discussion about the role of personality in forming supportive relationships, and in perceiving relationships as supportive. Furthermore, there have been suggestions that some types of support are effective for some types of stress but not others, and we do not yet know enough about the causal processes involved to be able to explain this (Gottlieb, 1983). For instance, although close relationships are usually protective, they can sometimes interfere with an adaptive mode of defence such as denial, which a person might be setting up in response to a particularly threatening event. Furthermore, adjustment to a new role in life may be best assisted by loose-knit networks, as when a mature woman leaves the domestic sphere to become a university student, or when adjusting to her newly divorced and single status. Given the complexities which have so far been uncovered, we may increasingly need to turn to experimental intervention research to better understand the mechanisms of support for differing types of stressful situations.

What kinds of intervention are suggested?

Intervention at either of two points in developing events could be justified: in event-producing situations and after an adverse event (see Figure 7.1). However, as suggested at the beginning of this chapter, the target group for the intervention should be particularly vulnerable in some way, that is, be predisposed biologically to a major psychiatric disorder, or be low in self-esteem, poor in coping skills, or low in support. The event must to some extent match this vulnerability, in that in the context of the person's past history, say, its interpretation poses a particularly marked threat.

A note of caution should be added. While the information assembled here facilitates the design and implementation of interventions that might reasonably be expected to be effective, chapter 9 shows that there is little firm evidence to demonstrate such effectiveness in many specific high-risk situations. Before serious thought can be given to designing general population interventions, there needs to be an accumulation of clear results from experimental targeted interventions for people coping with one particular life event or chronic strain. The following are examples of interventions which might be instituted in this way.

Intervention Point A: event-producing situations

I have argued so far that people who are highly likely to experience an event with implications severe enough to provoke a depressive illness can sometimes be identified. A history of failure in an area of life to which the person is highly committed not only makes him particularly vulnerable to depression following a further experience of failure, but can also raise the probability of further failures. A man with a poor employment history, who has lost several jobs and experienced intermittent phases of unemployment, has a considerably raised probability of becoming depressed when he is again made redundant (Eales, 1985), but will also have a raised chance of being near the top of an employer's list for redundancy in so far as it is the policy of many employers to exercise a 'last in first out' policy. It might be possible for people in such circumstances (perhaps when redundancies have been notified some weeks in advance) to be supported and perhaps taught techniques to cope with the anxiety and avoid being overpessimistic or 'catastrophising' (see next section). Other such opportunities might occur with people with recurring illness, or with couples considering divorce who have a long history of marital strife.

For people with long-standing difficult social circumstances that may throw up a crisis at any time, intervention might best combine practical help with a scheme to foster the person's sense of control over his or her life, to reduce their sense of hopelessness. Some kind of befriending scheme using volunteers would be a particularly promising approach, perhaps with people who have come through similarly difficult circumstances. Those with poor coping resources who might be particularly susceptible to depression may need to be helped to develop positive perceptions of their own capabilities and to lessen their perception of themselves as helpless and of low status. Social workers and other primary care workers are well placed to identify people who have long-term social difficulties and poor coping resources.

Those who have suffered from several episodes of schizophrenia are often less socially competent in managing their domestic and occupational affairs than they were before their illness. They are therefore likely to be more prone to experience adverse events associated with accommodation and employment, events which might precipitate a relapse. It might be possible to reduce risk if care was taken to ensure that, say, their landlady or employer was prepared to deal constructively with difficulties that arose, perhaps by involving a community psychiatric nurse as mediator. Placement support which at the least minimised the chances that the ex-patient would be evicted from his home or sacked from his job the first time a problem occurred would seem essential.

It has also been found that unanticipated events and changes are more likely to precipitate a relapse of schizophrenia than events for which the person is prepared. In a classic experiment reported in 1964, John Wing and his colleagues showed that long-stay schizophrenic patients given advance preparation for placements in an industrial rehabilitation unit were less likely to suffer a relapse than those who were unprepared.

An absence of information to aid the identification of those about to face a stressful event who would as a consequence be particularly susceptible to psychiatric disorder is obviously a good enough reason for not considering preventive intervention. However, if the cost of the intervention was small enough, it might actually be justifiable to mount a programme on a population level. For instance, a major operation, starting a new school and going on active military service are threatening events often known in advance of occurrence, but which only a small minority of people will find sufficiently distressing to make psychiatric disorder a likely consequence. However, the examples also have in common an institutional setting which provides a ready opportunity for mounting large-scale intervention and it may well be more cost-effective in these circumstances to provide a preventive programme for all experiencing the event. If children's anxiety in the transition to a new school can be eased by minimising the changes between class groups and between teachers at no extra cost, and no loss of educational effectiveness, it obviously makes sense to do so. If military training can incorporate an element of preparation for the emotional experience associated with active service abroad which prevents even a small number of psychiatric casualties, it may well also help to maintain the morale of others and be cost-effective in these terms. A simple leaflet routinely given out to patients before admission to hospital for common, straightforward operations, explaining the operation they are to undergo, common after-effects, the discomfort and temporary impairment of function likely to be experienced, and so on, may prove to be helpful in the sense of increasing feelings of control and might well aid their recovery. And for a very small number of patients it may also avert a psychiatric disorder. Of course, such a leaflet should be a supplement to, and not a substitute for, a one-to-one preparatory discussion between patient and doctor, and may be inappropriate for less straightforward procedures.

Intervention Point B: vulnerable people, after the event

The ideal model for intervention after a threatening event has occurred to a vulnerable person is that suggested by Parkes (1980) in his recommendations for bereavement counselling. His research on bereavement has led him to formulate a list of factors which make it possible to identify those likely to be at particular risk for psychiatric disorder. As described earlier, they include those who lack other supportive relationships, or whose previous relationship with the deceased has left them with an overwhelming sense of guilt, leading to self-punitive grief. Other circumstances predispose to the avoidance of grief including social pressures not to show emotion; a belief that they should, for instance, protect children from displays of grief; a fear of being thought to have broken down; or heavy use of tranquillisers to avoid the physiological accompaniments of grief. Given that a good deal is also known about how people successfully adapt to bereavement (Parkes and Weiss, 1983), a possible format for intervention programmes is already available. Intervention may be of a befriending nature, offering the person the opportunity to confide, and talk through his emotions, and gently guiding him towards a reassessment of his new position in life without the person he mourns. Or it may take a more structured approach drawn from cognitive therapy techniques.

Cognitive theorists like Beck have drawn attention to the tendency on the part of many who are depressed to interpret even quite minor, as well as more serious events, in terms of some negative self-perception. A friend failing to turn up for a date may reawaken deep-seated fears of abandonment. He argues that it is common for a depressed person to grossly exaggerate the negative implications of events (sometimes called 'catastrophising'): 'I didn't get that job – I'm not bright enough – I'll be unemployed or in low-level jobs for ever – I'll be bored and boring – my friends will abandon me – my husband won't love me any more.' Various types of cognitive therapy to bring an improvement in psychiatric disorders by altering maladaptive thinking appear to have been successful (Gelder, 1985).

Such maladaptive assumptions are a feature of depression itself, of course, and may not be present in the individual when he is not depressed. However, it is possible that cognitive changes occurring in the early stages of a depressive disorder may initiate a vicious circle that can transform an otherwise mild and short-lived reaction into one that is more severe and protracted. In this sense cognitive therapy might sometimes serve a preventive function. Furthermore, some of these sorts of approaches have been modified for more general use with those who are not already suffering a psychiatric disorder.

One technique involves helping a person to break down a problem into more manageable subproblems and consider the merits of various possible solutions to each part. After choosing a solution, a step-by-step plan of action is worked out. The value of each tactic is considered not just for the problem itself, but as an approach that might be used again on a future occasion so that the person can learn how better to cope with future problems (Gelder, 1985). McGuire and Sifneos (1970) describe the use of this approach for people who have recently experienced a serious loss of some kind – bereavement, redundancy at work, or divorce. Some stress management techniques for controlling anxiety, which have acquired a degree of popularity, also show certain similarities (e.g. Meichenbaum, 1977). These methods have, for instance, been shown to considerably reduce the symptoms of people who become unduly anxious before taking examinations (Meichenbaum, 1972).

If a person has a tendency to interpret events according to a particular negative cognitive schema, then this must be represented in some neurobiological code in the person's brain. And it seems that the biological state of an individual can undermine his perception of being able to cope – his level of fatigue, state of exhaustion or physical illness. This means that some attention to internal fatigue levels may also be of help in dealing with stress. Indeed, some hospitals have begun to experiment with providing complete physical rest as central to a treatment programme for cardiac cases, which is then followed by instruction on relaxation techniques through which people may be more effective in controlling anxiety (e.g. Charing Cross Hospital, London).

With most major life events, it is likely to be very difficult both to identify people who have recently experienced an event and find out which of them are likely to be susceptible to psychiatric disorder as a consequence. Although a wide range of mutual aid groups are now available, involving reciprocal aid among people who have in common one particular type of life stress, members typically only discover or are discovered by the organisation some considerable time after the event (Richardson and Goodman, 1983). Their support is then usually too late to avert psychiatric disorder as research is clear in showing that most disorder associated with life events develops quite rapidly after the event. However, many organisations could improve their preventive role by developing their out-reach methods and strengthening links with general practitioners and health visitors or other professional groups likely to have information on people currently facing those events. The Stillbirth and Neonatal Death Society in Britain, for instance, has produced an information package for hospitals to attempt both to encourage a more sensitive approach by hospital staff to the management of stillbirth cases (such as in disposing of the body) and to increase the chance that families will rapidly be put in touch with their organisation.

Perhaps the easiest, if not the earliest way to identify the people who are not coping with recent events is to wait until their distress brings them into contact with health or social services. The general practitioner is a first port of call for people with all manner of distressing circumstances. A good GP could provide preventive counselling. But where more intensive support is required, over a longer period, he or she needs to be able to put the patient into contact with a relevant mutual aid group, befriending scheme, counselling service, or psychiatric crisis support scheme.

Crisis intervention teams have developed as a part of statutory services in a number of areas in Britain. Clients are usually only referred to them, however, when they are already suffering serious psychiatric problems. Furthermore, people with a history of psychiatric disorder are more likely to be seen as suitable referrals by primary health care workers. These services are described in more detail in chapter 9.

Voluntary services, however, may sometimes be mobilised for people whose distress has not reached pathological proportions. The non-professional also has a number of advantages over professional services. They can avoid the role of help giver which casts the client into a dependent role. If they have experienced difficulties similar to the client, or live in a similar social environment, they are more likely to be able to foster the client's own coping skills and to achieve a friendship on equal terms. The principles of mutual aid are that members should be involved in a reciprocal supportive role. For this reason, Gottlieb (1983) argues that support schemes must avoid casting the non-professional into a professional type of mould and recreating the provider-client relationship.

However, a major difficulty in ensuring the effectiveness of any support scheme is to reach in time the small proportion of the population least able to cope with their crisis. Further work is needed to enable those specialist groups with support to offer to identify indicators of vulnerability and to find ways to reach their most needy group.

8
Approaches to prevention: macro-policies

There can be no doubt that an individual's psychological and personal social resources to a considerable extent determine his capacity to deal with many of the life events and difficulties he encounters. But adaptation is not solely dependent upon individual efforts, even if supported by close friends or relatives. There are also the wider influences of the society in which the person lives. The social and cultural environment provide constraints on a person's responses to events, influence his appraisal of events as stressful, and provide resources for dealing with them. Some patterns of behaviour, for example, are condemned, while others are highly valued. In western societies, it is not considered acceptable for a bereaved person to wander the streets wailing aloud, or for a man to seriously wound his wife's lover when he discovers the couple together.

The way in which people learn to make sense of what happens around them is deeply embedded in cultural assumptions. Social structures establish roles and statuses which have reciprocal responsibilities. The meaning to be attached to various social relationships is partly determined by such structures, the values which may motivate people, and the costs and benefits of various courses of action (Mechanic, 1986). Social roles contribute to a person's self-definition and motivation. Each role also carries social expectations, and opportunities or restrictions on functioning within the community. Some roles, for instance, require leadership, guidance and support for other community members, while others, such as the role of a sick person, offer an opportunity to avoid responsibility (Mechanic, 1986). Roles, like those associated with serious mental or physical disability, carry social stigma and exclusion and may negatively affect self-esteem, motivation and activity.

In terms of external resources for coping with life's difficulties, two of the most obvious, other than personal social support, are money and education. The social organisation of the community has important consequences for the distribution of such resources, and an individual's position within the social structure will therefore considerably affect his life chances. In some societies, boys are valued more than girls, and where resources are limited, this may produce differential nurturance. Advantage from birth in terms of income and parental education in modern societies continues to elevate the opportunities for survival, health, educational attainment, favourable occupation and privileged social position (Mechanic, 1986). And for people at all levels of competence, those launched from a position of greater social privilege tend to do better.

Many skills necessary for coping with challenges in the environment are taught formally in developed societies. Other learning takes place through informal channels and will to some extent be modified by the person's social position. However, social structures can change rapidly, sometimes because of sudden technological or economic developments. These have unstabilising effects on communities, as the transmission of effective coping skills inevitably to some extent lags behind.

Two aspects of social organisation provide the principal structure for daily activity through much of adult life – work and parenting. These roles have an important bearing on social status and financial resources, and both have been subject to rapid changes in many western countries in recent years.

The work role

For people working in a capitalist industrial society, paid employment will obviously to a large extent determine social status and resources. And, of course, it is not a straightforward either/or effect, those with jobs having status and resources, those without being dependent, and of low status. Many features of the job itself are also important. The status of various occupations is something which can be measured, and it is widely understood that managerial and professional occupations carry higher social status than manual work, and skilled manual work more than unskilled. It is a commonly used index in social research because of the extent to which it relates to a host of other social, economic and health variables.

People without paid employment, on the other hand, are without a potentially important source of self-esteem and a foothold on the status hierarchy. Unemployed people tend to be categorised in terms of the role they have lost, rather than a new role they have taken on. And often the implication is that it is in some measure their own fault that they are jobless. There are many people, including some health professionals, who consider that large numbers of the unemployed could get jobs if they wanted, and are choosing to be unemployed. A long series of eloquent articles on the health effects of unemployment, published in the *British Medical Journal* between November 1985 and February 1986, provoked correspondence along those lines (Smith, 1986c). Some people wrote to suggest that the unemployed should not reproduce and the young should be conscripted. It is possible that such stigmatising and victim-blaming attitudes are widespread – nobody wrote to take issue with those correspondents – and these attitudes inevitably help to make unemployment for some a humiliating and shameful experience.

Marie Jahoda (1979), after a lifetime of studying the unemployed, defines five reasons why employment is important to the individual beyond his or her requirement for financial support.

First among them is the fact that employment imposes a time structure on the waking day. Secondly, employment implies regularly shared experiences and contacts with people outside the family. Thirdly, employment links an individual to goals and purposes which transcend his own. Fourthly, employment defines aspects of status and identity. Finally, employment enforces activity.

Many studies confirm this appraisal.

Daniel's (1974) survey of 1,479 unemployed workers, for instance, found that, following concern about lack of money, respondents were most concerned about their boredom and lack of activity. The unattached young, in particular, were most likely to complain about restrictions imposed on their social mixing. The Economic Intelligence Unit (1982) also documented the effects of unemployment on the social lives of over a thousand unemployed people. While nearly half of those who had been without a job for up to eight weeks said they saw their friends as frequently as before, only a quarter of those unemployed for more than a year did so. Many unemployed people had difficulty in using their extra free time constructively. Nearly half watched more television (with a quarter watching four hours more per day), most believed retraining to be futile and in any case only 12 per cent had had any course suggested to them by Job Centres. Their fatalism was also clear in that only one in twenty expected to get another job within the next month, and only one in nine to do so within three months. Families of unemployed people also tend to be affected. Fagin (1981) describes how the wives of unemployed men often become depressed, and how their children may be affected in terms of changes in feeding and sleeping habits and in general behaviour.

Jahoda (1979) describes how many unemployed people actually decrease their use of clubs and free libraries, and reduce their reading. Budgeting, although more important, becomes progressively abandoned, and as time goes on family relations may deteriorate. Self-doubt, demoralisation, a lowered self-esteem and depressive moods reflect the impact of unemployment. Even among the normally most resilient, forward-looking and rebellious young people, resignation and restriction of ambition and desires were the rule (Jahoda, 1979).

Traditionally, a job has provided structure, social contact, goals, status and financial resources for life. Increasingly, however, people are finding themselves without a job for much of their lives. And even for those with jobs, the nature of employment has changed. A typical working life has decreased in years, and the working week in hours.

Unemployment and mental illness

Although the misery, shame, boredom, financial hardship, poor social life and low status associated with unemployment have been extensively documented, there have been disturbingly few careful longitudinal studies which have demonstrated that unemployment *causes* somatic or psychiatric disorder. Aggregate studies which compare the level of unemployment in a community over a given period with the death rate or the numbers of admissions to psychiatric hospitals for the same years, such as those conducted by Brenner, have many limitations and have been greatly criticised (see Miles, 1983). Brenner argued that the time lag between rises in unemployment during the period 1841 to 1971 and admissions to mental hospitals in New York State suggested a causal relationship (Brenner, 1973). However, such general measures cannot take account of other social

changes, or the changes which have taken place in psychiatric practice. And use of a slightly different time span might have produced
different results. In other words, crude comparisons do not enable
alternative explanations for correlations to be ruled out. A positive
relationship between mental hospital admissions and unemployment
may actually be reflecting the effects of poverty, rather than unemployment, on mental illness. Or it may even be that the mental
hospital admissions were employed people whose jobs became more
demanding during a recession.

There are many studies of this kind which report a positive correlation between unemployment and suicide (Platt, 1984). There is
similar evidence on parasuicide (non-fatal deliberate self-harm). Platt
and Kreitman (1984) show that the parasuicide rate in Edinburgh
was only once in the years 1976 to 1982 less than ten times higher
for unemployed men compared to men in jobs. For those unemployed
for longer than one year, the risk of parasuicide doubled. However,
the relationship was reduced in the year unemployment was highest,
and in the areas with the greatest unemployment, and it may be that
it is only highly stigmatising to be unemployed until unemployment
becomes very common in a particular group. After this point is
reached, misery, at least that associated with feelings of shame, is
reduced.

Cross-sectional studies – those which compare the health of a
group of employed people against that of a group of unemployed
people at one point in time – are even more limited in the information
they can provide on causation. A major methodological problem, of
course, is that poor health is often a cause of unemployment (rather
than vice versa), and poor health, physical or mental handicap reduces
a person's chances of obtaining a job when unemployed. This means
that comparisons between employed and unemployed persons which
fail to control for all the possible confounding factors will inevitably
find the unemployed to have poorer health. And in fact it is known
that unemployment does hit some groups more than others. Unemployed people are more likely to be unmarried, unskilled or semi-
skilled workers, able to earn comparatively low wages when employed,
and more likely to be very young, twice the otherwise expected
number of sixteen to nineteen-year-olds being without jobs (Moylem
and Davies, 1980). Fewer of the wives of unemployed men are
economically active than wives in general. Furthermore, as unskilled
jobs are hardest hit by the recession, and unskilled workers likely to

suffer worse health even when in work, the average unemployed person is likely to be less healthy than the average employee.

More important, from the point of view of establishing causation, are longitudinal studies which follow the same individuals over a period of time as their employment status changes. Unemployment may not have a serious deleterious effect on physical disorder (Smith, 1985), but the evidence that unemployment is sometimes the cause of suicide is overwhelming (Platt, 1984). It is increasingly clear, too, that it is a causal factor in depressive disorders. Banks and Jackson (1982) documented the effects of unemployment on school leavers over a twenty-month follow-up period. Their sample was first interviewed while still at school, at which time there were no differences in mental health ratings (using the GHQ) between those who subsequently found work and those who did not. On leaving school, however, ratings for the two groups diverged. Eales (1985), in a retrospective study of eighty unemployed men in London, was unusual in assessing health and employment status over time *and* rating mental status using clinical diagnostic criteria. One in seven of the men interviewed who were well at the time of job loss developed a relatively severe (case) affective disorder, and one in three a moderate or mild (borderline case) disorder. Most were depressive states arising soon after job loss. Feelings of shame were also reported by one in four men.

Bolton and Oatley (1987) interviewed forty-nine men who had just registered as unemployed and were seeking work at Job Centres in Brighton. They were aged between twenty and fifty-nine years and had become involuntarily unemployed less than two weeks previously after a full employment history. A matched sample of men in jobs was also obtained. Both groups were re-interviewed six to eight months later by which time fifteen unemployed men had found work. The ratings of depression at the two points in time showed no significant differences between employed and unemployed men at the first interview, but eight months later, the twenty men who had been continuously unemployed were considerably more depressed than they had been, and than other groups were. Some of them who had been well at the first interview scored above the threshold to be described as having a clinically significant depression on the Beck Depression Inventory (a self-rated questionnaire, Beck *et al.*, 1961).

Bolton and Oatley (1987) argue that the loss of a job has a causal role in depression inasmuch as the loss threatens the person's primary role through which they define their self-worth. They extend this explanation to the role of life events in general in the aetiology of depression. So they suggest that an adolescent becoming a drug addict can provoke depression in his parent if it threatens his or her feelings of self-worth as a good father or mother, and discovering a husband's affair can provoke depression in a woman if it threatens her perception of herself as a good wife. But depression will normally only occur when the person has no other roles which provide alternative sources of self-esteem, and if he or she lacks the resources to generate new ones.

A similar explanation for the finding that depression is most common among working-class women with three or more young children at home was put forward by Brown and Harris (1978). Two out of five such women were found to be depressed in any one year. They suggested that the presence of many children militated against the woman deriving satisfaction from her role as mother and acted as a constraint against her taking up activities outside the home where she might experience other role identities. If she was also without a close relationship with her husband or a job outside the home, she had few other potential sources of self-esteem and was therefore extremely vulnerable to depression.

Paid employment and social status have also been linked to the outcome of schizophrenia. With their limited ability to withstand stress, limited productive capacity and limited drive, many people with chronic schizophrenia in industrial societies not only suffer the stigma of mental illness but also experience further alienation through unemployment or menial jobs like dishwashing or envelope stuffing. Warner (1985) argues that the low social role, status and integration of people with schizophrenia strongly influences the course of their illnesses, and accounts for the better outcomes found in the non-industrial world compared to the west. From his cross-culutral review of the prevalence and course of schizophrenia, Warner shows that in the Third World people with schizophrenia are more readily returned to a useful working role, and frequently are much less stigmatised. Healing rituals encourage community involvement and aid reintegration, as well as generating optimism about recovery. Furthermore, family patterns of support in the Third World are better suited to the rehabilitation of the disorder. Family studies of psychotic patients in London and New York have found that about half the relatives are critical and demanding, whereas in North India this was true of fewer than one in five relatives (Leff *et al.*, 1987). This is likely to be a reflection of family patterns of interaction in general in the different cultures rather than specific to those with a mentally ill member. Warner (1985) concludes that in the Third World people with schizophrenia are more likely to retain their self-esteem, a feeling of value to the community, and a sense of belonging.

Warner suggests that the alienation of the schizophrenic person and his family in the west has its roots in the division of labour and the development of waged work. This might also explain the sex differences reported by many studies in recovery from schizophrenia. Following treatment for the disorder, many women return to an assured role as homemaker and experience less difficulty than people who must re-enter a competitive labour market. Finally, the effect of unemployment on schizophrenia may not only be the consequence of stigma and alienation, but it may also be linked to the lack of stimulation and activity which often characterises the experience of long-term unemployment. Wing and Brown (1970) linked the poverty of the daily existence typical of many back wards of the old mental asylums to negative features of the disorder, which could be improved by improved social care. However, many discharged patients who were unemployed and living at home and who were followed up by these investigators spent similar lengths of time doing nothing. It seems probable that lack of job opportunities can impede recovery from schizophrenia.

Occupational stress

The concept of social status has also frequently been used as an explanation for the differential health records of men in different types of job. For instance, Kahn and French (1962) found job status among blue-collar workers and supervisory personnel to have a substantial inverse relationship with their number of visits to the company dispensary in one large American organisation. A longitudinal study of men whose status changed through promotion or demotion confirmed that those who were promoted would get healthier and those demoted less healthy (see Kahn and French, 1970). Another study sought public opinion and evaluation of the jobs and the characteristics of two unknown men when the only information given to respondents was the job held by each man. Respondents tended to rate the status and prestige of jobs in the expected direction, but characteristics and evaluations of the jobs were also attributed to the job holders. A third-level manager was consistently rated as more ambitious, well-educated, skilled in administration, and hard-working than a low-skill craftsman. The investigators also found people holding those same sorts of jobs to have similar self-perceptions, so that job status and pay were positively related to self-esteem (see Kahn and French, 1970).

Of course, such correlations may not indicate a causal connection between job status and self-esteem. There has been a good deal of research on the nature and effects of occupational stress, but insufficient use of prospective designs to disentangle adequately the relative contribution of characteristics of the job and attributes, interests and motivation of the person (Kasl, 1984). Nevertheless, the view that role conflict could explain at least one common source of occupational stress became popular during the 1970s (Lofquist and Davis, 1969; Kahn and French, 1970). It was held that the threat to health arises not so much from characteristics of the job itself, but from an incompatibility of attributes of the person and the job or from conflicting aspects of the same role (e.g. House and Rizzo, 1972). When the demands of the job are found to be excessive, for instance, so that the person is caught between too many legitimate tasks, conflicts will arise. The work role may then also conflict with the person's other roles such as husband, wife or parent.

More straightforward links between jobs and stress have also been found. Common physiological indicators used include a raised heart rate, blood pressure, serum cortisol, corticosteroid and catecholamine levels. Kasl (1984) reviews sixteen studies linking these physiological indicators of stress with job characteristics. Those features of the job found to correlate with such variables included: external pacing of work demands (for example, where an employee must keep up with the fixed speed of the conveyor belt); tasks requiring a high level of continuous attention or vigilance; relatively drastic consequences of inadequate task performance; and psychological and physical constraints on the way the tasks were performed. Particularly stressful jobs in these respects are those done by sawmill workers and air traffic controllers. Studies of the physical health of air traffic controllers confirm this evaluation. Compared to workers in jobs of similar status without these features, air traffic controllers have a raised rate of hypertension, diabetes and peptic ulcer (see Kasl, 1984). Stressful work conditions often also lead people to adopt unhealthy coping responses, such as increasing their consumption of alcohol and tobacco and their propensity to take risks (Levi, 1979).

Most of the occupational stress research has dealt exclusively with men. Evidence on the health effects of occupational stress on women is scarce and research has hardly begun to look at the selection of factors which relate to working status (career goals, family finances) or at the conflicts which will inevitably be more common for women than men between paid employment and parenting (Kasl, 1984).

The role of parent

Despite the intrinsic rewards which most people assume to be conse-quent upon mothering, numerous authors have documented the high level of dissatisfaction among women engaged in full-time child care and housework (Oakley, 1974; Boulton, 1983) and others have noted that women at home with several very young children are particularly vulnerable to depression (Brown and Harris, 1978; Richman *et al.*, 1982; Pound and Mills, 1983). The unique stress of mothering seems to be at least partly due to its never-ending demands and constraints on activities unrelated to parenting. Mothers, as their role dictates in Britain and America, have sole responsibility for their children, and have responsibility for them all the time (Boulton, 1983).

The way responsibility for children falls heavily on one person is peculiar to our western industrial society. A cross-cultural study of mothering of pre-school children by Minturn and Lambert (1964) showed that the more usual pattern is for child rearing to be a shared role, mothers spending less than half their time in caring for their children. In most other societies, women combine child care with economic responsibilities. Children might go with their mothers to work in the field, men and women may work in groups with children playing around them so that they all supervise the children, or grand-mothers or older siblings may take responsibility while mothers carry out other tasks. Furthermore, families tend to live close together in large living units so that mothers are not socially isolated. This contrasts with western arrangements in which women live only with their nuclear families, often physically separated from other family members and other women and children. They remain outside the economic activities of the community and occupy a dependent role. Minturn and Lambert (1964) found that this arrangement was associated with less emotional stability in the way mothers dealt with their children, and less maternal warmth.

In her examination of the experience of mothering of fifty women in London, Boulton confirms the picture of high levels of distress associated with the role of caring for pre-school children. The study was of working-class and middle-class women who enjoyed basically good social conditions and who might be expected to find mothering rewarding. Two-thirds of the women did feel that their children brought their lives a sense of meaning and purpose but one-third did not, and only one in three women felt a sense of meaning and purpose *and* enjoyed looking after their children. Many more found the task of caring for their children irritating and frustrating. Their responses seemed to confirm Minturn and Lambert's claims that western arrangements are not as satisfactory as they might be. The women interviewed by Boulton felt physically and psychologically tied to their children, which limited their social contacts and activities. They felt outside the mainstream of society and socially and economically dependent on their husbands. Being segregated into separate households left them socially isolated from each other and the outside world. These frustrating and irritating features predominated over the pleasure they found in caring for their children.

How can society reduce role stress?

If evaluative systems operate within communities to influence self-esteem and physical and mental health according to roles and status, then two other social issues become relevant, in line with the reasoning of Mechanic (1970): (i) how does society attempt to develop the skills and competence of community members to prepare them to deal with the demands of their roles? (ii) what systems of rewards and punishments do organisations and communities develop in allocating roles and shaping role requirements?

(i) Education

The adequacy of preparation is a major determinant of whether or not, and to what degree, a situation is experienced as stressful. This can explain group differences, say, between more and less well-educated people in their ability to deal with authority, in that what people in different groups' experience as stress varies according to their differing preparatory systems. People frequently do well what they have been taught to do well, and areas of social incompetence can often be traced back to the inadequacy of preparatory institutions (Mechanic, 1970). Communities have to weigh up the costs and benefits of preparation from the perceived magnitude of the threat should training not be provided, the likelihood that skills can be acquired without training, the capacity to teach the skills and many other factors. Clearly the cost of human or machine error in putting a vessel into space is considered great enough to warrant formal preparations of personnel and machinery to cover every conceivable eventuality. Preparing adolescents for the potential difficulties of parenting does not, however, tip the balance in the same direction.

The educational background and subtle interpersonal skills which are central to personal effectiveness on an occupational and personal level are acquired partly through formal learning experiences in schools and partly informally through parents and peers. One identifiable societal response to promoting competence has been to attempt to compensate for disadvantages in informal networks by strengthening formal education. In Britain, the approach has been to provide schools serving disadvantaged communities with more resources so that they could offer lower teacher-pupil ratios and additional facilities (the Educational Priority Scheme). In the United States a more prominent intervention was perhaps the setting up of pre-school educational programmes for disadvantaged children.

Educationalists involved in the schemes have been highly optimistic about how they might be able to compensate for social inequalities and have often been disappointed in the outcome of programmes (e.g. Barnes, 1975). Many pre-school programmes were dropped when the impressive benefits from early evaluations of the Headstart projects seemed to have disappeared a few years later (Sylva, 1983), and scepticism replaced optimism. Some unexpected difficulties have been discovered, for instance, with the idea that it was easy to reach the target group by identifying priority areas where socially disadvantaged families were concentrated, and then concentrating resources in these geographical areas. Barnes (1975) quickly concluded that in fact most disadvantaged children are not in educational priority areas, and most children in educational priority areas are not disadvantaged. But some important lessons have now been learned, especially from the numerous evaluations of pre-school programmes in the United States.

Perhaps the most important lesson has been that educational practices which provide enriching experiences, extra tuition or other additional educational resources will have a limited impact if the experience ends at the school gates and the child returns to the same social and educational home environment each evening. It has now been shown that only by involving parents actively in the education of their children can lasting effects be achieved (Bronfenbrenner, 1975). In fact, the crucial role of parents in augmenting their children's educational gains is a message which educational researchers are increasingly emphasising. Hewison and Tizard (1980), for instance, show how involving parents by getting them to listen to their children read considerably improves the rate of acquisition of reading.

Bronfenbrenner (1975) examined seven pre-school projects serving poor black families in the US. Each project had collected evaluative information on the educational progress of participants compared to a similar sample of non-participants. Most of the data consisted of scores on intelligence tests and school achievement ratings. He found good evidence for some dramatic IQ gains during the year of the programme, but after graduation the children began to drop back towards where they would have been without the programme. In Bronfenbrenner's words, 'the substantial gains achieved in the first year of group intervention programmes tend to wash out once the programme is discontinued.'

But the seven projects were very different in format, and Bronfenbrenner found that if he looked separately at those programmes which were home-based rather than pre-school-based, the children involved made gains that held up three or four years later. He argued that it was not so much that the benefits came from the setting, but from the involvement of the parent as educator. He suggested that the programmes were helping to strengthen the emotional attachment between mother and child, increasing both the motivation of the child to learn from the mother and the responsiveness of the mother to the child. Because attachment behaviour is strongest at around two years of age, Bronfenbrenner argued that this kind of intervention is best mounted for two to three-year-olds. Programmes which are pre-school-based should come later, at age four to five years, so that they can prepare children for the school environment, but the parents' involvement should still be central. Once the child is at school, parental support should still be actively encouraged, in terms of showing an interest in the child's homework, and ensuring that effort is rewarded as much as achievement.

Like so many others who have documented the difficulties of providing preventive programmes, Bronfenbrenner also reports on the difficulties of reaching the most disadvantaged groups, and on how their disadvantage works against their deriving benefit from the service. Many poor mothers carry both breadwinning and child caring responsibilities unaided, which sap their physical and emotional energies. When they are so concerned with simple survival, they are not well placed to look favourably on schemes which demand both their time and their effort. Inevitably, Bronfenbrenner concludes that there are important political implications. Perhaps one parent could be freed from poverty-line income by paying her or him to stay with her or his children. Perhaps practical work with young children could be included in the school curriculum, such that hard-pushed parents could be helped and school children could gain an interest and experience in parenting.

Bronfenbrenner argues convincingly in favour of more family intervention of the type he showed to be most effective. He believes that not only does the target child derive long-term benefit, but gains are also extended to younger siblings through changes in the mother's attitude and behaviour, and are also experienced by the mother herself as she sees herself as a competent person capable of improving her own situation. A follow-up of some of the same children from the controlled studies some years later confirms many of Bronfenbrenner's conclusions. The Consortium for Longitudinal Studies (Lazar *et al.*, 1982) tracked down and reassessed many children involved in the same pre-school projects when they were aged between nine and nineteen years. They found most of the benefits that had been sustained to be definable in terms of parent support.

Each of the projects had differed so much that they were evaluated separately and treated as a series of independent replications and meticulously analysed. The team were able to demonstrate long-term benefits, but they were not the dramatic rises in IQ or substantial achievement gains that were originally anticipated. Rather, the projects seemed most effective in preventing school failure – project children were less likely to be kept down a year, or to be assigned to special or remedial classes, or to drop out of school.

On the surface, these benefits seemed unspectacular, but the details show impressive effects on children's attitudes and motivation and their parents' support for their efforts. Programme children showed a greater desire to achieve, and whatever their level of success, their mothers expressed more satisfaction with their children. Programme mothers also had higher aspirations for employment for their children. Lazar and colleagues (1982) suggested that programme children's enhanced motivation might be a reflection of their perceiving their parents' attitudes as a belief in and support of their efforts. They therefore saw the benefits of the projects as changing children from passive to active learners, and as making mothers more encouraging, such that they were able to bring about long-term gains in cognitive development.

(ii) Societal incentives

The adverse aspects of mothering have been described in terms of the isolated role of the parent who has sole full-time responsibility for her children, is outside the economic activities of the community, and occupies a dependent role and second-class status. Two quite opposite remedies have been proposed to enhance the esteem of mothers. The first, which has recently been forcefully argued by Leach (1979), suggests that strategies should be mounted to increase the status of motherhood in our society in relation to outside employment and thereby increase the potential for women to derive satisfaction, enjoyment and a sense of value from their role as full-time mothers. The second, which is the position taken by Boulton (1983), suggests instead that mother and children should be more fully integrated in the public sphere and that both men and women should share child rearing and economic roles.

The first proposal is based upon Leach's (1979) belief that child rearing has the potential to be as rewarding as the most demanding and interesting paid professions. But she argues that mothers who are unhappy in their role are inevitably advised to seek some outside employment rather than examining and attempting to change the circumstances that are depressing them. If she is 'stuck in all day' it is because there is nowhere for her to go with her baby; if she is lonely it might be because she has moved away from her friends and relatives. The solution does not have to be to seek paid employment. Leach argues in favour of providing the necessary financial resources to prevent mothers from being forced to seek outside employment; for planning resources and an environment to enable mothers to fulfil their role with a minimum of stress and a maximum of pleasure; to provide accessibility to information on child development to increase the interest of their job; and to educate the public to recognise the importance and status of child rearing.

Among Leach's suggestions are that many more public places should be provided where mothers and babies could meet socially during the day, such as the local-council-subsidised 'one o'clock clubs' in England. She also urges planners to take account of women with young children when designing the environment. Simple journeys to the shops can be daunting when pavements, doorways, escalators and even supermarket pay tills cannot easily be negotiated with a pushchair or pram plus toddler. But perhaps one of the worst hazards for mothers hoping to enjoy their role at home has arisen from the policy of replacing dilapidated terraced housing by blocks of flats. Not only are low-rise blocks often organised around stairwells that demand physical feats of mothers with babies and toddlers to negotiate, but they have seriously increased the social isolation of young families through their insensitive designs. Richman (1978) has argued that high-rise housing for mothers of young children explains some of the high incidence of maternal depression in her study of mothers in North London.

But Leach's suggestions would not change two of the fundamental disadvantages identified by Boulton, namely that women occupy a dependent role and that our economic organisation prohibits men from sharing a significant degree of the responsibility for child care. A large number of the middle-class women studied by Boulton were provided with many of the resources for enjoying motherhood that Leach sees as important, yet many were still frustrated and irritated by their role. They felt their own personality was submerged and that their children dominated their lives. An alternative solution is that women as well as men should have a role in productive work vital to society, and men as well as women share responsibility for their children (Boulton, 1983).

The means through which such changes might be achieved were formulated as long ago as 1966 by Gavron. As Boulton (1983) summarises them, the strategies include educating girls to prepare them for both family and employee roles; a recognition of fathers as sharers of active parenting; domestic work sharing on a principle of equity; supervised public play areas so that children may accompany adults in their public lives; attitude changes to recognise that figures other than the mother can be equally good child carers; greater priority in government policies to families; and restructuring work-places so that there are more part-time jobs, more job sharing, and flexible work arrangements.

In an ideal world one might want to make both sets of recommen-dations a reality, so that mothering, whether full- or part-time and when provided by the mother, father or other adult, is a rewarding, satisfying and enjoyable experience. If the quality of many mother-child relationships improved, not only might the self-esteem of mothers be enhanced, but, given the association between psychiatric disorder in mothers and behavioural problems in their children, it may also prove to be an important preventive strategy for children. Richman and her colleagues (1982) have demonstrated that early maternal depression is related to the later development of neurotic and anti-social symptoms in their children. They argue for preventive policies for the child's health aimed at mothers, strategies which would make it easier for them to do their job well and to derive pleasure and satisfaction from it. Pound and Mills (1983) note that few contemporary mothers had ever cared for a child before the arrival of their own first-born and have no knowledge of child care apart from their memories of their own childhood. They suggest that education for parenting should begin in school and continue over the early period of married life when people are facing the problems, and that small-scale mother and toddler groups should be fostered everywhere, groups which could provide companionship, emotional support and some covert education. Richman makes similar sugges-tions. Her other recommendations are familiar too: higher child benefit, more pre-school facilities, more direct support and advice from health visitors, housing policies which consider the physical and social needs of young families, improved environmental designs for pram pushers, and more flexible employment practices to allow both working mothers and fathers to fulfil their parenting role.

The recommendations which have been made in the literature for reducing occupational stress strike some similar chords, prevention being seen to be synonymous with improving the quality of working life and humanising the workplace (European Foundation, 1981). Lofquist and Davis (1969), for instance, maintain that this can best be done by employers through a careful consideration of the design of jobs, the design of the organisation, their recruitment procedures and the processes through which they go about resolving organisational problems. Beehr (1976) and Karasek (1979) identify the autonomy provided in the job as a particularly important moderator of occupational stress, and argue that jobs should be designed to maximise 'decision latitude'. In fact, Levi (1981) described recent efforts in Scandinavia to legislate to require employers to provide the worker with a significant amount of control over his or her job, together with some guarantees of job satisfaction.

Some companies provide counsellors in the workplace so that workers can discuss problems they encounter in their role. However, the counsellors rarely have the power to change the source of work difficulties and aim instead to help people adapt. Newman and Beehr (1979) review a number of experimental programmes in the workplace which provide training in interpersonal coping and in emotional defence strategies and positive thinking, and teach relaxation, meditation or physical fitness. However, good evaluative data on the effects of such approaches on the health of employees is lacking.

It has been suggested that organisations might be motivated to take the issue of occupational stress at least as seriously as they do the physical health and safety aspects of jobs in two ways. Firstly, substantial costs are associated with lost working days, and varying figures purporting to represent the scale of the loss to industry attributable to mental ill-health have been cited. While the precise validity of such calculations may be questionable, they invariably exceed estimated losses through strike action (MIND, 1971; C. L. Cooper, 1980). If evidence from controlled experimental studies could be accumulated to demonstrate reduced absenteeism, or an improved productivity during work time, the economic incentive for action would be overwhelming. Secondly, the legislation on health and safety at work could incorporate issues relating to psychological stress so that some measure of compulsion was available. Cooper (1980) reports that a number of successful disability claims in California have been based on occupational stress, and this has prompted a rapid growth of counselling services in the workplace. But despite detailed recommendations submitted by mental health organisations (MIND, 1971), the Robens Committee on Health and Safety at Work (Robens, 1972) almost completely omitted mental health issues from its report (Ennals, 1972).

While efforts can be made to improve the quality of parenting and occupational roles, this is rarely seen to be a viable approach towards reducing the deleterious effects of unemployment. This is because it is a non-role. There is no feature, other than signing on or looking for jobs, which requires activity or provides social contact that can be enhanced. Approaches to reducing associated distress must inevitably involve the creation of a role, probably one allied to the occupational role, such that the individual becomes a contributing rather than dependent member of the community again.

Reducing unemployment is the most obvious way to attack the problem. The Charter for Jobs (1985) produced by a consortium of managers and professionals from all major political parties in London has put forward specific proposals for increasing employment. They include placing greater priority on the completion of labour-intensive projects (building roads, perhaps) and a reduction in the employer's national insurance contribution to reduce the cost of labour without reducing wages.

An alternative is to share out existing jobs more equally, perhaps by employing two people to do one job between them. Many public organisations now permit this. Often it is married women with children who take up these opportunities, but there have also been similar initiatives for school leavers (see Smith, 1986b). Shorter working weeks and working days, and earlier retirement ages, would also share jobs more widely.

Socially useful jobs can be created by providing subsidies to organisations which would otherwise not be able to fund the position. This is the basis of Britain's community programme mounted by the Manpower Services Commission. The Charter for Jobs proposes that all Britain's 1.25 million long-term unemployed be guaranteed a job on such a programme.

Finally, education and training opportunities can be increased to reduce the numbers of unemployed people and provide a temporary alternative role as student or trainee. This is how the Manpower Services Commission has opted to spend the biggest part of its budget. Its training schemes for young people aim to provide a bridge between school and work, to prepare them for the labour market, create a more efficient workforce, and provide work experience. Opportunities for vocational education and training in Britain are, however, markedly fewer than those provided in the United States, Japan and West Germany (see Smith, 1986a).

There is evidence that the provision of meaningful activity to structure the day and provide social contact is protective against depression among the unemployed. Hepworth (1980) found that among the unemployed men she interviewed, the single best predictor of psychiatric problems (as assessed by the GHQ) was whether or not the person felt his time was occupied. Breakwell and colleagues (1982) report that the nineteen young people who completed a Manpower Services Commission's Introduction to Work Scheme (three days' work experience, two days' training in college) had better self-esteem than 112 unemployed young people of similar socioeconomic and educational backgrounds, despite the fact that the former were highly critical of the scheme. A larger-scale study by Stafford (1982) showed training schemes to have a protective effect. The general mental health (GHQ) of over 1,000 young people was assessed before they left school. Some months later the GHQs of those who got jobs had improved, while there was a significant deterioration for those who became unemployed, and no significant change for those going on to youth training schemes. The beneficial effects of the training scheme in these terms were, however, temporary. Ex-trainees who found jobs compared to ex-trainees who became unemployed showed divergent health ratings on re-interview some months later.

Even with the increasing numbers of such schemes, it is clear that for many years to come a large number of people will spend considerable lengths of time unemployed. In the absence of an occupational role, other interpersonal roles may become crucial sources of self-esteem. Gore (1978) found that unemployed men with family and friendship ties which were perceived as supportive, which afforded a high level of social activity outside the house, and which provided a perceived opportunity to discuss problems had fewer depressive symptoms than men losing their jobs at the same time who had less social support. Bolton and Oatley (1987) also found the amount of social contact available to the unemployed men when they lost their jobs was related to depressive symptoms eight months later. The men in whom the greatest increase in depression scores occurred were described as having few or no friends, and having a narrow range of social contacts almost exclusively confined to the family. Bolton and Oatley (1987) argue that the importance of these relationships is that they provide a role within which a person can experience himself as worthwhile. However, given that it seems that the quantity rather than quality of relationships was of most importance (contrary to the findings on protective factors against depression in women where quality is paramount), their protective effect may also be attributable to the opportunities for activity they provide. The implications of such findings are that it may be possible to forge new social networks among the workforce of an industry facing closure or severe cutbacks before employees are made redundant, through social gatherings, meetings or discussion groups, which can be maintained in unemployment. And community activities which facilitate friendships between unemployed people and provide sporting, social or occupational activities may be helpful.

Finally, if long-term unemployment is likely to be a reality for many people, it may become desirable to reduce people's commitment to the employed role and to attempt more vigorously to reduce the stigma of unemployment. Bolton and Oatley (1987) found that unemployed men who rose regularly each morning were more likely than men with more relaxed habits to secure new jobs, which was seen to be indicative of a self-motivated personality and resourcefulness. But people who are highly committed to finding work who do not manage to secure jobs suffer considerably lower psychological well-being (Warr, 1984, p. 274). The less palatable logic of this finding would suggest that high commitment to the employed role needs to be reduced when probability of finding work is almost negligible. Appropriate strategies for individuals depend on the economic state and policies of the society and the likelihood that individuals' efforts can secure them jobs.

Conclusions

When Marie Jahoda put together her five features of paid employment important for the health and welfare of the individual, she might equally have applied it to any of our primary roles. People need a sense of identity and status within a subgroup or culture from a role which requires their active involvement, provides structure to the working day, provides goals which transcend their own, and provides the opportunity for social contact. The extent that people can obtain these requirements from their primary role, be it worker, parent, student, homemaker or keen amateur darts player, will be related to the presence of depressive symptomatology and recovery from serious psychiatric disorder.

Social organisations can do much to promote role satisfaction, and to provide new roles. The effectiveness of societal approaches is often mediated by long-term changes brought about in the individual's psychosocial environment. Short-term changes have only short-term benefits. This is best illustrated in the role of preparatory educational processes. The contribution of both formal institutions such as schools and informal networks such as parents and peers was discussed in earlier paragraphs. Attempts to reduce disadvantage in terms of poor performance in schools through intensive but temporary formal compensatory programmes showed the benefits to be equally temporary. Involving parents in compensatory programmes, however, achieved long-term changes to the child's psychosocial environment and long-term educational and social benefits. Similarly, training schemes for unemployed people only afford health benefits equal to an occupational role for as long as the scheme lasts.

9
Preventive interventions

There are serious methodological problems associated with attempting to evaluate preventive programmes in terms of reductions in the incidence of specific psychiatric disorders. The constraints of time and money are perhaps the most obvious. A programme which aims to improve parent-child relationships as a preventive measure for adult depression, say, cannot be adequately assessed in these terms until twenty or more years later when the experimental group would be expected to have developed fewer episodes of depression than a matched comparison group. Obviously a great deal will happen to all the individuals concerned during this interval, events which will not be subject to the control of the researchers but will undoubtedly influence the probability that the individuals will be vulnerable to depression. And the cost of keeping track of a sample over so many years would be prohibitive. Not surprisingly, those setting up and evaluating preventive programmes almost always choose other methods. Effectiveness of a programme is usually assessed in the weeks, months and sometimes a few years after the completion of the intervention. This means that either a different outcome measure is needed by which it can be judged as successful (raised self-esteem, self-efficacy, or warmth of parent-child relationship, say), or the programme must be aimed at a group who are highly likely to develop a psychiatric disorder in the very near future, recently bereaved persons perhaps. These are, in fact, the two most common types of preventive programme.

There have been other types of preventive programme too, of course. There have been efforts, for instance, to modify the environmental cause of stress, such as in the transition from primary to secondary school, and attempts to maximise people's sense of control over their own lives in circumstances in which they commonly feel helpless, such as when living in residential homes for the elderly. Each of these sorts of approaches can justifiably be expected to have some preventive benefits, given the aetiological research reviewed in early chapters, although without the selection of a high-risk group evidence of their effectiveness can be expected to be attenuated (see chapter 7).

The projects to be described have been categorised into vulnerability-focused projects and event-centred interventions. Most of the first category are in fact programmes aimed at augmenting the coping skills or resilience of young children. Some have attempted to do so by working directly with children, others by work with mothers. There have been some similar approaches (aimed at enhancing coping skills) with adults. The general heading of vulnerability-focused intervention also includes some innovative approaches to reducing the vulnerability of people with a history of serious psychiatric illness to further acute episodes of disorder.

Studies (not great in number) aiming to reduce the psychiatric sequelae of life events have been placed in a second section. Some approaches have involved advance preparation for events, while others have provided counselling support after an event.

The projects described all aim to modify factors which have been shown to have some aetiological significance in the development of psychiatric disorder, or aim to help individuals known to be at high risk of disorder. Unfortunately, most can be criticised. Indeed, the seriousness of the problem is indicated by the fact that some of the best studies in prevention are reviewed here and their shortcomings therefore highlight the general low level of methodological sophistication of most studies in the field. However, it is all too easy to criticise – and in fact, the major difficulty has been not so much with a poor standard of research as in the complex way a range of causal factors interact and accumulate to produce mental illness, and the very real difficulties of untangling their relative effects. Perhaps even more important is that although we may now know a good deal about who is at risk and why, much less is known about how to bring about desired changes. This is not only apparent from experimental research projects, but also from the health service practices which have preventive functions. Three service areas have had declared preventive aims: community mental health centres, primary care services, and psychiatric services concerned with preventing relapse, particularly through crisis intervention methods. A third section of this chapter will provide a rough sketch of the professional services with a preventive responsibility at the present time, and how and with what success they achieve their aims.

I Vulnerability-focused experimental intervention

(i) School-based programmes for young children

Most child-centred preventive programmes have been directed at young, socially disadvantaged children who may also be showing early signs of disturbed behaviour. The aims have usually been to reduce disturbed behaviour and increase coping skills, that is, the child's problem-solving ability, concentration, persistence, or social skills perhaps. By this means it has usually been hoped that there would be long-term benefits across a range of potential psychiatric disorders. However, in addition to these broad-based approaches, there have been some (rare) projects focusing on the prevention of a particular disorder, such as Mednick and his colleagues' efforts to prevent schizophrenia.

Mednick and his colleagues (1981b) conducted skin conductance tests on 1,800 three-year-olds living in Mauritius. Early research had shown that deviant scores in children in terms of autonomic nervous system recovery responsiveness predicted to some extent later schizophrenia. Children with particularly deviant scores were selected for the intervention programme. Half of the selected 200 high-risk children were given a special nursery school education of three years' duration aiming to increase their positive social interactions. The remainder served as a community comparison group. Just before the children started primary school, assessments of their behaviour during free play sessions were made. Four children at a time, who were unfamiliar to each other, were brought together in an unfamiliar playroom with new toys. An observer coded each child's behaviour according to the amount of time spent watching, playing constructively alone, or interacting positively with the other children. The high-risk children who had been educated in nursery schools spent more time than the comparison group in social interactive play, while the comparison group spent more time in constructive play. Whether the achievement of this rather limited goal will have a long-term effect on the incidence of schizophrenia will have to await the outcome of future follow-up enquiries. Further follow-ups of each of the different groups should reveal not only whether the intervention has been effective but also whether or not the simple physiological test used was indeed an accurate predictor of schizophrenia.

As described in the preceding chapter, there have been many attempts to provide compensatory education for disadvantaged preschool children. A pertinent factor related to the effectiveness of such efforts has been the extent of parental involvement in the programmes. There has been speculation that this was because the active support of the parent ensured some continuity of relevant stimulation and perhaps also enhanced the parent-child relationship, effects which lasted well beyond the cessation of the special programme. None the less, many preventive programmes aiming to augment children's coping skills in an attempt to prevent adjustment problems have often not involved parents. Despite this, some report impressive effects.

Shure and Spivack (1982) have developed a training programme over a number of years designed to improve the 'interpersonal cognitive problem solving skills' (ICPS) of young children. The aim was to help disadvantaged children think through and solve interpersonal problems and so reduce aberrant impulsive or inhibited behaviour before they entered the primary grades at school. In an evaluation of the programme, children were taught a range of skills over an eight-week period in a pre-school educational setting to enable them to play games focusing on listening to and observing others, and learning that they have thoughts, feelings and motives in problem situations. The games were then incorporated into the school curriculum for a training time involving twelve weeks of formal scripted sessions, once during the nursery year and again during the kindergarten year.

The evaluation examined the ICPS skills and the classroom behaviour of 113 black inner-city low-socio-economic-status four to five-year-olds before and after training in the nursery year and again in the kindergarten year. A comparison group of children matched on age, sex, intelligence and initial ICPS test scores and behavioural characteristics was also assessed at the same time. The ICPS measurements were based on the child's answers to questions like how he would obtain a toy from a classmate, and what he would expect to happen next in a game sequence in which an object had been taken from an adult without permission.

The children given the training were found to make greater gains in ICPS scores than comparison children and their behavioural adjustment was also superior. Over the two-year study period, well-adjusted children given the training were less likely to begin showing behavioural difficulties than well-adjusted children in the comparison group, and aberrant behaviours when present were less likely to persist. The investigators argue that the approach therefore has important implications for prevention through building coping skills in high-risk children. From their own and other similar investigations, they believe trained children are likely to show more flexible responses to interpersonal problem situations, trying more than one way to solve a problem, not give up too quickly and retreat after failure, and to apply solutions likely to have a positive effect on others. However, in reviewing the evidence on the effectiveness of a number of similar such training programmes, Durlak and Jason (1984) report that other investigators using the Shure and Spivack approach have either failed to obtain positive effects, or have noted that if adjustment had improved, it did not correlate with gains in problem-solving ability. The approach seems intuitively appealing, and there has been enthusiasm for introducing the technique into school curriculae (Durlak and Jason, 1984). Its effectiveness as a preventive strategy in the long term, however, remains unclear.

Another well-known American school-based intervention programme is the Primary Mental Health Project in Rochester, New York (described in Durlak and Jason, 1984). Mass screening for early indications of school maladjustment identifies a high-risk group and these are provided with a behavioural or relationship-oriented training by paraprofessionals (such as trained volunteers, students, housewives or counsellors). The children are seen in groups during the school day but outside normal classroom sessions for one hour per week. If a behavioural programme is being used, individual treatment goals are developed for each child, involving the reinforcement of positive social behaviour in terms of the school setting. For 'acting-out' children this might mean rewarding behaviour such as waiting their turn, listening to others, or following directions. Evaluations conducted in at least fifteen different school districts have indicated that such prompt attention to early-detected dysfunction is effective in improving the behaviour of young children at school and that enhanced adjustment has by and large been maintained for the period of evaluation which has ranged from a few weeks to several years. Given that childhood behaviour problems frequently persist

into adulthood, this method may have considerable preventive potential and is relatively inexpensive to provide on a population basis.
Follow-ups of these children in future years can be expected to
reveal its long-term effects.

A modification of this approach in public schools in Detroit trained
both pre-school children and their parents (Rickel *et al.*, 1984).
Parents were given training sessions at the school in such behaviours
as talking and listening to the child, commenting positively on desired
behaviour, expressing anger, and conflict resolution and discipline.
Again, differences between children given the programme and a
matched comparison group were demonstrated, and were still present
two years later. Programme children achieved similar levels of matu-
ration in cognitive and social-emotional development to a low-risk
comparison group who had not experienced behavioural or learning
difficulties. Both teams of investigators (Rickel and colleagues, and
Durlak and colleagues) are so convinced of the merits of such
approaches, even in the absence of long-term evidence, that they
already advocate their routine implementation in schools.

Strikingly positive results have been produced from a research
project of a similar nature in England. One thousand junior school
children of seven years and 3,000 seniors aged eleven to twelve
years in Newcastle were screened to identify children with emerging
psychiatric and educational difficulties (Kolvin *et al.*, 1981). The
265 high-risk juniors and 309 maladjusted seniors were randomly
allocated to an untreated comparison group or to one of three types
of intervention: for juniors, there was a 'nurture' group, playgroup
or parent counselling-teacher support group and for seniors, a behaviour therapy, group therapy or parent counselling-teacher support
group. The psychotherapeutic intervention (discussion groups for
seniors and playgroups for children) and behaviour therapy had the
most marked effects. These were also the least expensive and shortest
programmes of the six: 3 months (one school term) of group therapy,
twenty weeks of behaviour therapy. Furthermore, follow-ups after
eighteen months and three years showed that on a range of clinical
outcome measures and indices of improvement, the positive effects
(compared to the no treatment group) seemed to increase with time
even though the intervention had ceased.

The psychotherapeutic methods were based on the ideas of Carl
Rogers. Six trained social workers held discussion sessions for seventeen groups of four or five same-sex senior children, and playgroup

sessions for seventeen groups of four or five mixed-sex juniors, within the ordinary school setting. Then sessions of forty minutes for each group were held over a three-month period. Such techniques require considerable specialised training for therapists who aim to establish warm, accepting relationships with group members, but direct play or discussion as little as possible, respecting the child's ability to solve his own problems. The junior group were supplied with toys for creative play: dolls, puppets, dressing-up clothes, plasticine and toy cars. The behaviour therapy involved training from a psychologist for thirty-nine teachers of seventy-two children (amongst their ordinary classes) in the use of social reinforcement. The method used systematic and contingent teacher praise, attention and approval. Occasionally material or concrete rewards were also used.

Kolvin and his colleagues were surprised at the success of the school-based interventions and, in line with American experiences, conclude that such approaches should be widely instituted in schools, perhaps by redeploying some of the staffing resources of existing child guidance or child psychiatric services.

(ii) Home-based programmes for young children and their families

There have also been attempts to provide professional intervention programmes for high-risk children in their own homes. Despite Bronfenbrenner's (1975) conclusions that home-based programmes for pre-school children were more likely to have long-term effects than school-based programmes, at least two carefully evaluated programmes that have worked with families produced disappointing results. The parent counselling-teacher support programmes mounted by Kolvin and his colleagues (1981), for instance, were the least effective and most expensive of the different methods of intervention that they tried. Social workers kept teachers informed about home circumstances and encouraged contact between teacher and parent. They provided parents with information about the child's work at school, encouraged the parent to ask about and praise the child for appropriate behaviour or achievement, and provided direct social work help for family problems. The intervention produced only marginally better clinical outcomes and improvements than occurred spontaneously within the no treatment comparison group.

Johnson and Breckenridge (1982) evaluated a programme aimed at low-income Mexican American families in Houston whose financial, language and ethnic group problems were added to by having moved away from prior support systems like the extended family. The parent-child development programme was expensive, involving about 500 hours of training over a two-year period for families with one to three-year-olds. It aimed to prepare economically disadvantaged children to enter school with cognitive and social skills that would reduce their potential disadvantage in school. Parents and siblings were offered English language classes, and mothers were visited at home to help them become more aware of their child's language and cognitive development and emotional state. Later, mothers attended group discussions on child management, which the investigators had previously demonstrated to be an effective programme in terms of increasing the expression of affection by the mother towards the child. The study reported by them in 1982 was to see if these practices brought about the intended preventive effect, namely a reduction in behaviour problems in the children.

Child behaviour was assessed from interviews with mothers when the programme children and a non-intervention comparison group were an average five and a half years old. The boys who had not been involved in the programme were significantly more destructive, overactive, negative-attention-seeking and less emotionally sensitive than boys who had participated and than girls whether or not they participated. But there was no evidence of benefit to the girls, although the investigators optimistically suggest that benefits may not be apparent until some years later.

However, the families involved in these intervention programmes tend to have multiple social problems and often parental psychiatric problems. They are frequently dependent on professional social services to solve their problems for them. It is probable that such interventions offering yet more professional advice and support have been less effective than they might have been because they have not succeeded in getting parents to take more responsibility and a more active, problem-solving role towards their own social difficulties and towards improving the behaviour and development of their children. A rather different sort of approach is likely to be needed to bring about such changes. A helpful approach might be one which recognises that mothers with psychiatric problems of their own will need support to bolster their own self-esteem and coping skills before they in turn can offer better support to their children. One source of improved self-esteem, of course, is to experience success in bringing about improvements in the child's behaviour or development. But to gain such rewards, they must see themselves as the crucial change-agents – not teachers, social workers or psychologists.

There are two particularly promising interventions in these terms, which are also considerably less expensive programmes than those just described: voluntary befriending schemes, and intensive, well-structured health visiting for mothers of high-risk young children. Homestart, a community-based scheme of family support, was set up in Leicester in 1973 and has since spread to many other towns in the United Kingdom and stimulated other similar befriending projects. Inspired by research which has shown the powerful effects on the child's development of the mother's parenting style and feelings of control in her role, the aim was to focus on the mother as model and home teacher for her child (Eyken, 1982). The most appropriate target group, however, was disadvantaged families with many children whose circumstances frequently threatened to overwhelm the mother in her struggle for survival, and prevailed against her giving each child much individual attention. Often she also developed a sense of powerlessness and low self-regard. The parents were not, therefore, seen merely as 'change-agents', but as people in their own right who might need help, who could only be expected to participate in a scheme in which volunteers came to their own homes to help and support them according to their needs. The project was based on the use of volunteers in a 'mum-to-mum' relationship, aiming to build up the parent's self-confidence, to help her to find stimulating and enjoyable activities to do with her children, to use local resources like playgroups and the toy library, and derive pleasure and a sense of competence in her role.

Over the four-year evaluation period, families were most often referred to the project by social workers and health visitors. All were socially disadvantaged. Two out of five were single mothers, and most were on a very low income. Of the 303 families referred to the project between 1974 and 1978, 226 were matched with a Homestart volunteer. Fifty of the client families, with 132 children between them, had children who were either on the At Risk register, on supervision orders, or otherwise stated to be at risk of coming into institutional care.

The benefits of the scheme have not been demonstrated by use of a comparison group, but have been described in a detailed description of its operation over a four-year period by Willem van der

Eyken. For instance, only eighteen of the 132 children did end up in substitute care during the four years, and the Homestart organiser judged two-thirds of the 156 families whose befriending had ceased or been ongoing for more than a year to have undergone considerable change for the better, and only 8 per cent to have shown no change. The possibility that the organiser might show a favourable bias in judgment was not confirmed from assessments of some of the same families by social workers and health visitors. In fact, the organiser was considerably more pessimistic than they were in her assessments of benefit. 'Change' tended to mean different things for different families, but may have meant, for instance, that a mother who had been under pressure from her environment, children, and poverty had been rehoused, had obtained part-time employment, and found pre-school placements for her children, and had a noticeably more positive and relaxed attitude towards her children (Eyken, 1982). After Homestart involvement, twenty-seven (of 156) families no longer required social work input, twenty-five families were rehoused, nine parents split up, eleven were married, nine mothers found jobs and six became volunteers for Homestart. Although these changes cannot be attributed directly to the intervention, without any indication of what might have occurred in its absence, the assessments of professionals, volunteers and the families themselves seemed to suggest that a good deal of these changes were brought about or facilitated by the scheme. Eyken argues that such material changes inevitably reflect attitudinal shifts within the family, changes in the quality of relationships with the children, and improvements in the self-esteem of the parents.

It was also argued that the Homestart volunteers were often able to offer much more stable support for the mothers than social workers, not least because of the frequent rapid turnover of the latter. Seventy-five of the seventy-seven volunteers who joined the project more than one year before January 1978 actually were continuing their befriending on that date. Most gave between two and six hours a week over to their Homestart activities (home visits, phone calls to doctors, schools and families, letters, meetings and so on) and befriended from one to three families. This unusually high commitment from volunteers was attributed by Eyken to the recruitment procedures, which effectively weeded out people unwilling to put in too much time by demanding a full-day training commitment at the outset, and by the support provided by the organisation.

A similar befriending organisation, Newpin, offering friendship, support and practical assistance, exists in South London, and has also been subject to some evaluation. A major aim was to reduce the high incidence of maternal depression, child abuse and neglect (Pound *et al.*, 1985). Volunteers were recruited from the local community, trained part-time for twelve weeks, and then paired with client mothers referred by social workers, health visitors or family doctors. Mothers were usually referred because of isolation, depression or problems in parenting. The pair formed a contract for their relationship. Volunteers visited client mothers, often several times a week, and encouraged them to go with them to the project drop-in centre with their children for training sessions and social meetings with other mothers. The contract would terminate by mutual agreement after a number of weeks when the presenting problem was agreed to be resolved or when the client had made wider social contacts.

A notable aspect of the work was that the volunteers lived in similar circumstances and came from backgrounds almost as deprived as client mothers. They were expected to offer whatever help they thought was needed, and friendship and support to enable the client to broaden her social contacts and to seek the help she needed to resolve her difficulties. The pilot study of a dozen volunteer-client pairs showed that the benefits of the friendships were felt by volunteers as well as clients. Almost all clients and volunteers had made new friends and every one of them had someone with whom they confided at a deep level (Pound *et al.*, 1985). The evaluation was based on self-reports, and therefore open to bias, but was nevertheless impressive in its own terms. Nineteen of the twenty-four women felt they had learned to understand people better, seventeen said their confidence and self-esteem had improved, and difficulties with their husbands or cohabitees and wider family had been reduced.

The women came from backgrounds known to be associated with a high rate of depression. Ten of the eleven referrals had been separated from one or both parents in childhood, eight had three or more changes of main caretaker in the early years, nine had been deserted by husbands or cohabitees during pregnancy or shortly after, and finance and housing problems were almost universal. It is for this reason that even relatively small effects in such a group of women would be impressive. Such women tend to have a great deal of chronic depressive disorder which often proves difficult for general practitioners to treat. Moreover, an improvement in the mother's psychological health would be likely to have a beneficial effect on her children. Mills and her colleagues (1985), in an observational study of depressed and non-depressed women with their children, found that children of depressed women made fewer verbal approaches to their mothers, and depressed mothers linked into and extended their child's talk or play less than non-depressed mothers. This poor meshing between the depressed mother and her child may go some way towards explaining poorer cognitive development and greater likelihood of behavioural disturbance among such children (see Richman *et al.*, 1982). Informal observations of mothers and their children in the Newpin befriending group led Pound and Mills (1983) to believe that the women's relationship with her children were better than in an 'untreated' and less disadvantaged neighbouring group of mothers.

Another impressive family intervention programme has used health visitors to support mothers in designing and carrying out stimulating and rewarding educational tasks with their children (Child Development Project, 1984). Eighty-six health visitors in six disadvantaged areas of England, Wales and Eire, randomly allocated to intervention or comparison groups, participated in the experimental health visiting scheme. Up to twenty month-old children were randomly selected from the caseloads of the health visitors, involving in all over 1,000 families. Visitors were trained to modify their usual directive approach, and work out with the parent, as equal partners, how best to help the child. Many families lived in run-down unsuitable housing blocks, many mothers had experienced several bouts of depression, often starting from the birth of a child, and financial difficulties were common, as was reliance on junk food and dependence on welfare services. Mothers often had little faith in themselves as competent parents and saw professionals as having the controlling power over their lives. Hence the aim of the health visitor was to foster self-reliance rather than reliance and dependence on professionals. They spent one hour every month for twenty months working in the home with the parent. They would talk about the child's recent progress and whether and with what success the child had completed the activities worked out at the last visit. A cartoon illustration of a common child management problem and a possible solution was also discussed.

The developmental levels of the children, the quality of parent-child relationship, and of the home environments were assessed by trained interviewers at the beginning, middle and end of the intervention phase. The Child Developmental Programme has yet to produce a full evaluation, but from the first year's comparisons the intervention appears to have considerably improved the home environment in terms of socioeducational level (presence of books, intellectual activities, educational aspirations), language, and cognitive content (thinking and problem-solving activities given). A variety of statistical analyses planned on the most recent data will reveal the effect on a range of other factors, including maternal self-esteem, diet and child social and activity levels (Child Development Project, 1984).

One final example of a preventive project focusing on the young child's home life has been instituted for children who have been placed in foster care. When a suitable placement has been found, it is important to minimise the possibility of a further breakdown in the child's relationship with his or her caretakers. Between 200,000 and 500,000 children have been reported to be in foster care at any one time in the United States, and placement failures are far from uncommon (Schaeffer et al., 1982). Schaeffer and colleagues have described their attempts to provide an experimental psychotherapeutic programme of crisis intervention with fostered children aiming to prevent such failures with the accompanying 'bouncing' of children with progressively more difficult behavioural reactions and damaged self-esteem.

(iii) Promoting personal control in adults

People who are able to plan their lives, or who deal in a positive way with events which threaten their well-being and their aspirations, are more likely to avoid becoming trapped into unsatisfactory lifestyles and consequent high levels of stress (Quinton and Rutter, 1983; Harris et al., 1987b). By contrast, those who tend to see themselves as in the hands of fate or powerful others are both more prone to adverse events and less likely to cope well (Johnson and Sarason, 1978). Helplessness has been argued to be an antecedent factor in the development of depression (Seligman, 1975; Harris et al., 1987b). If only for this reason, there is some justification for claiming that the efforts of voluntary groups which campaign for higher status for their client groups are potentially preventive of depression. For instance, many women's groups aim to help women to become more aware of their rights, to see themselves in a more positive light, to become more active, assertive and independent rather than passive or helpless. Some offer courses of assertion training (e.g. Potter, Lee and West, 1979). A similar approach can sometimes be seen in groups aiming to promote the best interests of homosexual people or people from ethnic minorities, especially in their aims of consciousness raising. However, there has been little, if any, research that has monitored the effects of such programmes either on assertiveness itself or psychiatric disorder.

The befriending and health visiting programmes described in the preceding section may also serve to reduce helpless attitudes and foster a sense of control in disadvantaged and isolated mothers. Of course, an inability to look forward, to concentrate and to take an interest in what he or she is doing or supposed to do, and a general sense of helplessness, are also common symptoms of clinical depression. Tableman and her colleagues (1982) mounted a stress management training scheme to try to enhance practical coping skills among women showing such symptoms. These low-income women in Ionia County, Michigan, were offered ten weekly sessions in groups of six to twelve, each lasting two and a half to three hours. Another random sample was not offered training and served as a comparison group. Three of the group sessions were devoted to enhancing self-esteem and identifying stress-producing aspects of social relationships; five covered life planning, accepting responsibility and techniques for taking control; two explored stress and stress management techniques including relaxation. Trained women were found to have made greater improvements than the comparison group in mental health status, using Cornell Index Scores, between the initial interview and follow-up interview three months after completing the course.

Many of the women who were clients of the befriending schemes or chosen as subjects of stress management training schemes found themselves, through a long chain of adverse circumstances, poor planning and poor coping, in chronically difficult social circumstances which they felt powerless to influence. However, similar feelings of powerlessness might arise quite differently, say, through increasing physical incapacity from old age or newly acquired disability. Over a relatively short period of time, many elderly people find themselves incapable of managing to live independently and need to move into supported accommodation. From managing their own financial affairs, buying and preparing their own meals, determining their physical environment, and structuring their daily routine, they may find such opportunities to exercise personal control are no longer available. It is now well documented that a decline in health, alertness and activity often occurs in elderly people after entering nursing homes (Rodin, 1983).

Rodin (1983) has conducted an extensive literature review and two experimental studies on the effects of increasing the perceived control of residents of supported homes for the elderly. Her review led her to expect that a lack of control contributed to psychological withdrawal, physical disease or deterioration, and even death. Indeed, she argues that the degree of biologically mandated decline with aging has been overestimated because environmental and personal events associated with old age so commonly produce a loss of control (Rodin, 1985). An early study trained carers to encourage elderly residents of a convalescent home to make a greater number of choices and to become more responsible for making daily decisions. Residents were told they could determine what their rooms looked like, where and when they would like to go out, and who they wanted to spend time with. On a different floor of the same home, although in theory the same options were available, a second group of residents were treated in the more customary way, and encouraged to feel that the staff would care for them and try to satisfy their needs. The group given greater responsibility became more active and alert than the second group, and engaged in many different kinds of activity such as going to the cinema and seeking out new friends. From a physician's blind evaluation of the residents' medical records, it was found that the 'responsible' residents also showed greater improvements in health during the six months following the intervention. Most impressive of all were the different death rates. After eighteen months, 15 per cent of the intervention group and 30 per cent of the comparison group died (see Rodin, 1983).

A second study by the same investigators took a more structured approach and used stress training methods developed by Meichenbaum (1977) to enhance the perceived control of nursing home residents in their management of everyday stresses (Rodin, 1983). This involved an educational phase to communicate the idea to residents that events in themselves were not responsible for the stress experienced, but rather it was their own thoughts and feelings towards the event which brought anxiety or depression. They were made explicitly aware of their own forms of negative self-statements. In the second week they were taught new self-statements to encourage a more realistic appraisal of adverse events, help them to generate alternative solutions and to exert control. These skills were practised in the third week.

Forty residents were randomly assigned to one of four groups – a trained group, a group who spent an equal amount of time with the researcher, but just chatting, a third treated as in the first study and simply instructed to take more responsibility in decision making, and a fourth who were given no special treatment at all.

Before training began, each resident was given a one-hour interview during which they were rated according to the choices they currently exercised, and the amount of decision making they would like to have. Their daily activities were directly observed, and they were questioned about what they did both inside and outside the home. Their health was rated both from self-ratings of eyesight, appetite, memory, energy, sleeping difficulty and depression, and from the assessments of the staff physician. There were also other questions about the frequency with which they encountered fifty problems commonly experienced by residents in nursing homes, and how bothersome or distressing they found each of them, from which actual and perceived stress was assessed.

The measures were repeated one month after the intervention programme ended. In all outcome measures, the specially trained group showed superior health, with the no treatment group always showing the worst, and the other two groups having comparable and intermediate effects. The trained group felt more in control and engaged in more active behaviour, they showed an increased ability to modify problem situations and decreased their use of tranquillisers and sleeping pills while the three other groups increased theirs. Furthermore, a re-examination of medical records eighteen months later showed a range of illnesses, diseases and deaths had occurred in the interim. Three residents died, five developed illnesses requiring hospitalisation, and ten developed a new or a decline in a chronic condition. Only one of these illnesses (one case of Paget's disease) had affected a member of the self-instructional group, and none of them had died.

Increasing the control institutional residents have over their lives does not necessarily require complex or specialist educational

resources. Schulz (1976) showed that visits by college undergrad-
uates to nursing home patients had a much greater benefit in terms
of self-rated happiness and feeling useful, and in terms of several
ratings of health, activity and use of medication, if the timing and
length of visits were determined by the patient. If the visits were at
fixed times so that the patient knew when they would occur, they
were also found to be helpful, but random visits, although enjoyed,
were not more beneficial than no visits at all. A disturbing insight
from this research was gained from the effect on those visited of the
cessation of the programme. Two years later, not only was the health
of the groups who had found visits beneficial showing a greater
decline than that of other groups, but effects were also reflected in
mortality rates, showing that it is crucial that positive interventions
are not introduced and then withdrawn.

(iv) Reducing vulnerability to relapse

A consistent picture has emerged from the research on the course
of schizophrenia, of an optimum socioemotional environment that
enables an optimum level of functioning and a minimum risk of
relapse. Conditions which are grossly understimulating will promote
withdrawal and regression. Rapid social changes, arousing environmental events and pressure from overcritical or overprotective relatives can lead to acute disturbance. There is evidence that changes
to both aspects of the environment of those with a history of schizophrenia can greatly reduce their risk of relapse with florid symptoms,
especially when combined with maintenance neuroleptics, which are
independently effective.

For instance, the work which revealed 'expressed emotion' (EE)
in the family home to be linked to the patient's risk of relapse (see
chapter 5) has stimulated several experimental preventive
programmes (see Barrowclough and Tarrier, 1984, for a review).
Leff and his colleagues (1982) attempted to identify relatives with a
high rate of expressed emotion (EE) and change their styles of
interacting or reduce the amount of time they spent together. They
provided educational sessions in the hospital for groups of relatives,
whether rated high or low on EE. Families were taught about the
nature, course and treatment of schizophrenia, and that many of
their relative's irritating or distressing behaviours were symptoms
of his illness. They were advised that the patient was particularly

susceptible to new events, and to prepare him or her well in advance of unavoidable changes, and to avoid criticism and overinvolvement as much as possible. Relatives were also expected to gain insight into better ways of relating to the patient from discussions in groups with both low and high EE members about how to handle specific problems that commonly occurred. Families were also visited in their own homes when they could be seen with the patient, and a form of family therapy used, with the same aims in mind as the educational sessions.

The results showed that high levels of criticism were reduced in about half the high EE relatives, and overinvolvement in slightly fewer. Of twenty-four ex-patients with high EE relatives, of whom twelve had been randomly selected for the intervention group while the other twelve served as comparisons, a total of seven relapsed within nine months. Six of the seven were in the comparison group. The only experimental patient to relapse was one for whom the researchers had been unable to reduce either EE or face-to-face contact with the relative. Two years later, the benefits were still apparent (Leff et al., 1985). Of the patients who remained on medication throughout the two-year period, seven of the nine comparison sample relapsed (78 per cent) and only two of the ten experimental patients (20 per cent). However, two other experimental patients committed suicide, which increases the failure rate to 40 per cent in the experimental group. Both suicides were patients whose relatives remained high on EE. Three comparison group patients also attempted suicide, but unsuccessfully. Finally, the protective effect of medication was most graphically illustrated by the five patients who stopped taking it during the two-year period. Four relapsed, three within a month of stopping medication, the fourth four months later. The patient who remained well was a woman living with her sister, who had spontaneously changed from high to low EE during the first few months after the patient's discharge.

Similar reductions in relapse rates have been achieved by at least four other groups of investigators working with families (Leff et al., 1985). One other programme which has been evaluated over a two-year period is that by Falloon and his colleagues (1985) in America. Relapse of patients remaining on medication was 83 per cent in the comparison group and 12 per cent in the experimental group. Like Leff's team, they emphasise the importance of continued medication, especially for those patients in high-risk situations. Falloon and his colleagues, however, also lay stress on the possibilities in family therapy for enhancing the quality of life of the ex-patient and his family, and for improving his or her long-term social functioning.

Another highly acclaimed innovative programme is the community living scheme in Madison, Wisconsin, developed by Test and Stein (1978). It was presented as an alternative to traditional hospital care. Patients were housed in their own locality, but not necessarily in the homes of family or friends. Many were provided with treatment and rehabilitation in the hospital on a daily basis. Time in hospital was gradually reduced, and after a work skills training, help was given in seeking open employment. Patients with stabilised but chronic severe psychoses were then followed so closely in the community that a relapse of florid symptoms could almost be eliminated. They were watched and helped in their own neighbourhood as closely as they might be on many hospital wards. Test and Stein, a social worker and psychiatrist, ensured that a member of the mental health staff was available twenty-four hours a day, seven days a week, to help chronic patients learn to shop, cater and budget for themselves, find work, and settle housing, employment and other crises. They were helped to make good use of their leisure time, and support was also provided, where appropriate, to the family. The outcome of this intensive programme of community support was assessed by comparing patients randomly assigned to the programme with those receiving routine mental health centre care (which treated almost all patients in hospital in the first instance). At the end of a year, the rates of readmission to hospital were 6 per cent for clients of the community programme, and 58 per cent for clients of routine mental health centre care. The former group also had fewer symptoms, greater self-esteem, and were more satisfied with their lives. This was achieved without shifting the care to the family. The support given aimed to avoid rehospitalisation or a return to the home of a relative. However, in order to maintain patients in their own homes, it was essential that psychotic behaviour was brought very rapidly under control, and the method was therefore heavily reliant on methods of rapid tranquillisation to deal with emerging acute episodes of disorder.

This programme shows that patients can be successfully treated *and* continue to live in the community, and that the cycle of recurrent relapse and readmission to hospital can be broken. Patients functioned better, given this intensive support – but only as long as the support lasted. When after fourteen months they were transferred back to routine mental health centre care, the clinical condition and social functioning of many of the patients deteriorated, so that after a few months they were faring as poorly as those who had received routine care all along.

II Event-centred intervention

Supporting people through stressful transitions

It is now widely accepted by mental health workers that distressing events can provoke a depressive illness or precipitate other kinds of mental or physical disorder in vulnerable people. It is also known that there is good evidence, as reviewed in a previous chapter, that social support can be in some way protective. These two findings have been used to justify a whole range of supportive interventions for people in distressing circumstances. Unfortunately, most interventions have not been based on an accurate understanding of the kinds of events and the qualities of social support that might bring about important effects, or the kinds of circumstances which might render a person likely to respond adversely. Events such as marital separation and transition to secondary school, sometimes selected as stressful events, will not necessarily pose any great threat to mental health. A husband or wife who is leaving to set up home with a new partner will not be likely to be experiencing the same degree of threat as the spouse he or she is leaving unsupported. Children moving on to secondary school with their best friend and living in supportive, caring family homes will probably not find the experience too distressing. Mutual aid groups for bereaved people may not necessarily provide the most important aspects of support and some interventions will offer support to people who already are supported by more important relationships than those offered.

Such qualitative issues tend to be ignored by many of those who have mounted preventive programmes, who take a health-predicting rather than a disease-modelling approach (see chapter 3). For instance, Bloom and his colleagues (1982) designed a support programme for a typical cross-section of newly separated people of both sexes, rather than selecting from them a particularly vulnerable group. They offered the services of a counsellor, available for regular assistance over the six-month period, and the opportunity to participate in a number of study groups looking at problems like career planning and employment prospects, legal and financial issues, single parenting problems, housing and homemaking, and socialisation and personal self-esteem. But not only were subjects not preselected as being at high risk for psychiatric illness, it was also found that among those offered the intervention programme, those who took up the offer had *lower* initial anxiety scores and were more aware of the problems associated with separation than those who did not partici- pate. It is therefore quite possible that participants were not a particu- larly vulnerable group at all, and those most in need of help did not receive it, a common finding of social researchers. Reported psychological problems and symptom checklist scores on neuras- thenia and anxiety dropped significantly for the experimental group over the six-month study period, but not for the comparison group. It is questionable, however, whether any serious psychiatric sequelae were prevented. As Bloom observes, future programmes would need to place greater weight on a 'proactive outreach role' to involve those who were coping less adequately.

A more accessible sample of people facing a highly threatening event is provided by those admitted to hospital for essential surgery for life-threatening illnesses. Maguire and his colleagues (1980) offered counselling and practical advice to women undergoing mastectomy following a diagnosis of breast cancer. But this study also failed to take account of differences in the circumstances of the study sample which would make some of them more vulnerable to psychiatric disorder than others. It would not be surprising if coun- selling had limited preventive benefits if the woman was married to a very supportive husband, whereas to a woman straining to keep her marriage intact, whose spouse was intermittently meeting with another woman, a perceived loss of sexual attractiveness might pose a considerable threat, and counselling may have a more important effect.

A specially trained nurse saw patients before and after their oper- ation and discussed with them their feelings about losing a breast, and demonstrated the use of a range of external breast prostheses. After the patient was discharged from hospital, the nurse visited her every two months to check arm movements, to encourage the woman to do the recommended exercises, and to talk about the woman's relationship with her sexual partner, her feelings about breast loss, and to encourage her to return to work and/or become socially active again.

A total of 152 women were randomly assigned for counselling or to a comparison group. Symptoms of anxiety or depression and the occurrence of sexual problems were rated shortly before the operation and three, twelve and eighteen months later. Equal numbers in both groups suffered from an episode of morbid anxiety or depression, or experienced marked sexual problems at some stage over the two-year follow-up period. However, episodes of depression and anxiety lasted an average of six months among counselled women but did not clear up on average for over ten months among the comparison group. Furthermore, counselled women showed a superior social adjustment, return to work, adaptation to breast loss, and satisfaction with breast prosthesis (Maguire *et al.*, 1983).

Despite these obvious benefits of the programme, which may well have been even more marked had subjects been considered separately according to the extent to which they were supported by their sexual partner, Maguire and his colleagues conclude that it was *not* a successful preventive programme, because the reduced duration of psychiatric problems was at least partly attributable to the early detection of psychiatric symptoms and prompt referral for treatment.

Other examples of general approaches to helping people adapt to worrying and distressing events can be found in abundance in the voluntary sector in the mutual aid or self-help movement. Self-help directories list hundreds of groups around Britain (see, for example, *The Sunday Times Directory*, Gillie *et al.*, 1982), such as Alateen to help twelve to twenty-year-olds overcome problems associated with having an alcoholic family member; Compassionate Friends, for bereaved parents; the Royal National Institute for the Blind; MENCAP, for parents of mentally handicapped children; and MIND, the National Association for Mental Health. They have been defined by Richardson and Goodman (1983) as 'groups of people who feel they have a common problem and have joined together to try to do something about it'. A more detailed classification according to function is difficult, as Richardson and Goodman found, because even in mutual aid groups established for people with ostensibly the same problem, individual members will have differing definitions of the nature of their problem and may be seeking very different types of solution. One of the significant characteristics of mutual aid is that it can perform a number of functions, and have a number of purposes and activities at the same time (Richardson and Goodman, 1983). They may have any or all of five basic functions: emotional support, information and advice, direct services, social activities and pressure group activities.

Preventing mental illness is rarely specified as one of their aims, however, even though emotional support is the function most commonly associated with them, and in practice, relatively few of their activities are oriented towards prevention. Some organisations rarely, if ever, have self-help face-to-face group meetings between members with common difficulties. Furthermore, it appears from the evaluation by Richardson and Goodman (1983) that most people join self-help or mutual aid groups only after they have worked through their feelings of loss and grief associated with the crisis. Only one-third of widows belonging to the National Association of Widows (NAW) joined within twelve months of bereavement, and over half the membership of MENCAP (for parents of mentally handicapped children) and NCSWD (for carers of elderly dependants) joined only after five years or more of caring. They may therefore be more appropriately described as coping strategies for people with chronic difficulties. Members joined for advice, information, and to campaign to improve the situation for other people with their problem.

This means that they cannot, on the whole, be considered as preventive strategies in terms of a pathological response to the initial crisis, although they may be protective in terms of providing a supportive resource in the event of future crises. They may help members to feel more in control of their problems, with access to information, advice and practical assistance if required, and some make close personal friendships from which they can derive consider-able support. Both of these might prove to be protective in future crises and even help to make crises less likely to occur.

It was argued in chapter 7 that there were two optimum points of intervention in relation to crises if event-related psychiatric disorders were to be prevented. The first (intervention point A) was before a predictable event, or in circumstances highly likely to result in a threatening life event. The approach might include facilitating antici-patory coping, changes to the circumstances to reduce the probability of the event occurring, or changes in the dynamics of the event such that it becomes less threatening. The second (intervention point B) was after the event and after it had become possible to identify those people in whom it was particularly likely to provoke a psychiatric disorder.

(i) Intervention point A

Both Wolfer and Visintainer (1979) and Ferguson (1979) have demonstrated that preparing young children and their mothers for the admission of the child to hospital for a tonsillectomy reduced the child's fears and anxiety and uncooperative behaviour during pre-surgical preparation, and problem behaviour after discharge from hospital. Both studies also found that the youngest children (three to four year-olds) were most upset by the pre-operative stages whatever the form of preparation (and whether or not it was helpful).

Wolfer and Visintainer compared five different approaches to preparing the children and their mothers, involving various combinations of pre-hospital information (booklet, hospital play kit), information after admission, and continuity of care from one responsible nurse. All forms of preparation were found to help make the experience less distressing than for children in a control group receiving no special information and normal changes of nursing staff. The greatest benefits were demonstrated, however, for those receiving the information at home before admission *and* either of the special treatments in hospital, nursing support or additional information. This also reduced anxiety among the mothers. Ferguson (1979) evaluated two other methods, a fifteen-minute film show after admission and a pre-admission home visit. The film showed two children going to have their tonsils out, worried at first, but becoming confident after preparation. The home visit was from a nurse who also met the child personally on admission and cared for him thereafter. She gave the child and his mother as much information about the hospital and the operation as possible. Both methods proved beneficial but the film was most helpful to the youngest children, and probably more appropriate to their level of verbal skills and understanding.

There have been, in fact, a large number of projects in which investigators have attempted to prevent the anxiety and pain associated with medical and dental procedures (see Peterson and Brownlee-Duffeck, 1984; and Johnson, 1984, for instance). Some studies have reported that individuals with a defensive attitude of denial or avoidance, who prefer to understand as little as possible of the surgical procedures, do not necessarily benefit from anticipatory guidance. However Peterson and Brownlee-Duffeck conclude that in most cases and for most conditions, children and adults benefit from preparation. Johnson (1984) concluded that information about how the patient was likely to feel *after* the operation, and practical advice on how to help his or her own recovery, through, say particular exercises, was beneficial. Her review, and her own research with adult gastroendoscopy patients, showed a high level of agreement that this kind of pre-operative information can in some way reduce fear, pain, length of hospitalisation, and in general speed recovery. She argues that intervention is helpful if it enhances the patient's feelings of control, rather than provides extensive details of operative procedures. The increased predictability of events, pains, discomforts and setbacks, and greater feelings of self-efficacy in being able to deal with them, leads to less distress. An unpredicted event, or much greater pain than expected, on the other hand, may lead the patient to believe things are not going as they should be and therefore increase his or her anxiety. It seems probable, however, that individual differences in the desire for behavioural involvement in one's own health care will contribute to the beneficial effects of an increased opportunity to do so (Rodin, 1985).

To some extent, many such programmes may be missing the more fundamental source of threat in hospitalisation and surgery which is relevant to preventing psychiatric sequelae rather than enhancing physical recovery. Parental separation is frequently mentioned as the principal cause of anxiety in hospitalised children, and relatively little documented evidence exists of the effects of preparing the child for the separation, or enabling parents to have a more direct supportive role during hospital treatment (Peterson and Brownlee-Duffeck, 1984). In many surgical operations for adults, the most threatening element may well be the long-term significance of the operation (such as in vasectomy, mastectomy, loss of limb, cancer). Anticipatory guidance remains a promising, but unproved preventive strategy, at least as regards depression.

A different kind of preventive approach involves modifying the environmental source of anxiety. In starting a new secondary school, for instance, a good deal of anxiety may result from the new organisational arrangement in which each child moves from one classroom to another several times a day, to a different teacher each time, and often a different peer group. Felner and his colleagues (1982) mounted an experimental organisational change for students starting high school. A random sample of new students were assigned to one of four classes who stayed together for four basic academic subjects. Their 'homeroom' teachers maintained a high level of contact with them and were the primary liaison between school and parents. Other new pupils, who formed a comparison group, were dispersed more widely and attended classes with a constantly shifting peer group. The comparison group showed signs of academic and personal difficulties associated with the change of school over the first year, which did not happen for the experimental group. Academic adjustment, the perception by the students of the general social environment, their self-concept and attendance, rated at the beginning and end of their first year, all showed significant differences between the two groups. Because a decline in academic performance and an increase in absenteeism are factors associated with school problems and drop-out, Felner argues that this low-cost intervention effectively reduces the risk of future school difficulties.

(ii) Intervention point B

On the whole, only a small proportion of people experiencing a major threatening life event will develop psychiatric disorder of any kind. Follow-up studies of people who experience a particular type of event enable an examination of the circumstances under which they are most likely to do so, and therefore allow a preventive programme to be directed specifically at this relatively high-risk group.

Research on bereavement has progressed through these stages. Parkes (1975) followed up a sample of widows and widowers in Boston for twelve months, from which he derived a list of predictive factors which could be assessed at the time of bereavement and which were correlated with poor outcome a year later. They included clinging behaviour towards the dying patient, angry or self-reproachful behaviour, being unprepared for the patient's death, lack of a supportive family, low socioeconomic status, and an intuitive guess by staff nursing the dying patient that the relatives would cope badly. These factors were incorporated into a predictive questionnaire through which Parkes was able to categorise bereaved persons as at high or low risk of psychiatric disorder.

Parkes (1981) evaluated the Family Services of St Christopher's Hospice for the dying in London, which used trained volunteer counsellors to visit relatives at home. Although details of visits and the time period over which visits took place were not supplied, the paper implies that volunteers also had a befriending role suggestive of a number of visits over an extended period. Relatives identified as at high risk of psychiatric disorder from the predictive question-naire were randomly allocated to one of two groups, an experimental group (thirty-two people) offered the counselling, or a comparison group (thirty-five people) who were not. The supported group had fewer, and less serious autonomic symptoms and a lower consump-tion of drugs, alcohol and tobacco than the comparison group twenty months after bereavement.

Similarly, Raphael (1977) used a questionnaire to determine risk according to the extent to which bereaved persons saw their families as unsupportive, the bereavement traumatic, their marriage ambi-valent, and their life complicated by crises other than the bereave-ment. In this way she selected sixty-four widows from a total of 194 as being at high risk of psychiatric disorder and randomly selected half of them for counselling support. Between one and nine lengthy counselling sessions by herself (a psychiatrist) were provided in the client's own home over a three-month period after bereavement. A marked difference was found between the supported and unsup-ported group thirteen months after bereavement on a checklist of fifty-seven symptoms which commonly take people to a doctor. The difference was greatest amongst those who had been rated as having a high level of perceived non-supportiveness in their social network during the crisis. Among these individuals, fourteen out of sixteen had a good outcome (i.e. few psychiatric symptoms) if counselled compared to only two out of fourteen who did not receive counselling. Both Parkes (1981) and Raphael (1977) also followed up a number of low-risk relatives who proved to have similar health ratings to the high-risk supported group. Both investigators maintained that the intervention effectively reduced the risk status of the high-risk group to the level of bereaved relatives initially assessed as being at low risk of psychiatric disorder.

Preventive programmes like these might be greatly appreciated by a large proportion of people experiencing this sort of traumatic event. But the programme can be demonstrated as effective in terms of 'hard' criteria only by focusing on a selected high-risk group and offering relevant, high-quality support. As has been argued in earlier sections and has been borne out by Parkes's review of other bereavement counselling efforts, many investigators have failed to select a high-risk group. Furthermore, some have offered intervention as long as six months after the bereavement and provided telephone therapy or sporadic, poorly planned visiting (Parkes, 1980). Not surprisingly they were unable to show preventive benefits.

Prevention within statutory services

The foregoing descriptions of projects represent a handful from an extensive literature. Some of those which seem concordant with the theoretical perspective of this book have been described in some detail. They would seem to support the contention that at present key concepts in effective prevention must include the enhancement of self-esteem and a personal sense of control over the prevailing or potential adverse circumstances and events in one's life, or one's response to uncontrollable events, and the provision of appropriate social support and social skill training in augmenting such attributes and working through natural emotions aroused by events. And it is clear that it is often possible to distinguish those people (from the circumstances of their lives) who would benefit from such help from those who have adequate resources and are more resilient to adversity.

How do these issues relate to current practice? What existing services might be seen as having some role in prevention? Can they be judged to be having any success?

(i) American community mental health centres

At no time has there been an explicitly stated concern for prevention and commitment to funding preventive services on such a scale as when President Kennedy announced his comprehensive community mental health centre programme in 1963. Each American state was to designate catchment areas serving between 75,000 and 200,000 people which would be served by a CMHC, and each centre would provide preventive, as well as a full range of therapeutic services (Levine, 1981). Nearly twenty years later the emphasis on prevention was reaffirmed in the Mental Health Systems Act of 1980. This legislation followed recommendations by President Carter's Commission on Mental Health, which was assisted in its work by the reports produced by thirty-five Task Panels. These Task Panel

reports ranged widely in length and quality, but the report on prevention was one of the more cohesive and creative efforts. Even so, it
failed to mention the paucity of convincing evidence to demonstrate
the long-range efficacy of many preventive programmes (Levine,
1981). Many of the Task Panel's recommendations were reflected
in the President's Commission's report, and the legislation which
followed.

The Task Panel on prevention suggested a focus on helping to
reduce the stressful effects of life crises like unemployment, retirement, bereavement and marital disruption; and examining the nature
of social environments (hospitals, schools), with the intention of
creating healthier environments in which people might achieve their
full potential. It was argued that preventive activities should be aimed
at all age groups, but the first priority should be interventions that
might prevent children from developing disorder in later life (Glasscote, 1980).

Despite President Kennedy's call for prevention to be a fundamental component of the work of the CMHCs, most, in practice,
neglected this area. Prevention fell within the consultation and
education category, on which only 5 per cent of funds could be
expended and which in any case included work other than prevention
(Roberts and Peterson, 1984). A survey by the Joint Information
Service of the preventive activities taking place in CMHCs under
the relevant federal support programme showed that, with a few
exceptions, prevention was a marginal activity if it featured at all
(Glasscote, 1980). Such work that was done was often carried out
by paraprofessionals for whom funding arrangements were tenuous.
Programmes consisted of public education about potentially
hazardous or healthy pursuits, or programmes aiming to educate and
support people in their efforts to cope with stressful transitions.
However, out of the 390 centres included in the survey in 1977, only
a handful were judged to have substantial programmes consistent
with the notion of primary prevention (Glasscote, 1980). Among
these few, the problems encountered in setting up and managing the
programmes had been substantial.

Six CMHCs were chosen by Glasscote's team as having a greater
commitment than most to preventive programming, and these were
studied in more detail. The sorts of programmes available included
divorce workshops which may, for instance, have involved a residential weekend experience for the family to help parents be more aware

of the effects of their action on the children. They also found support groups for the newly single/divorced/bereaved, groups for 'entrapped housewives' and their children, and sessions for parents of difficult/ delinquent teenagers. Other provision was primarily educational. There were classes for the general public, but aimed at particular groups, such as the newly married, single parents, parents, the aged, depressed women, potential alcoholics or potential child abusers. There was also self-assertion training, couples courses, and 'understanding aging' courses. But although they were seen to be addressing important problems experienced by distressed people, and although some had done surveys of satisfaction of participants showing involvement to be judged beneficial, no evaluation had been conducted to provide any objective evidence that the programmes had prevented anything (Glasscote, 1980). It seems that although some CMHCs have begun to devise programmes with preventive goals, many of the projects have foundered. And a disappointing lack of information has been collected on the success or failure of their efforts.

(ii) British primary care services

Professionals with direct contact with the community have a responsibility to detect difficulties at the earliest stage in their development and to be vigilant for risk situations where problems are likely to develop. In this sense they are seen as having a role to play in prevention. A social worker visiting a large family where the husband had recently lost his job would be expected to be on the look-out for a range of problems which could arise from the financial hardship and extra emotional strains put on the family, and to support and advise the family accordingly. If difficulties began to escalate and there were signs that either parent was becoming depressed and not coping, then there would be a need for social work support to try to head off further problems.

General practitioners have a responsibility to immunise children against communicable diseases, to be vigilant for developmental problems, to advise on healthy lifestyles including smoking, drinking and diet, and to screen high-risk groups for possible disease (by cervical smears or blood pressure tests for example). As the Royal College of General Practitioners (1972) stated, the GP is supposed to intervene 'educationally, preventively and therapeutically to promote his patients' health'. Teachers are expected to recognise and respond to learning difficulties and together with education welfare officers and educational psychologists help to prevent emotional problems and school drop-out. Community psychiatric nurses are expected to help prevent a recurrence of mental illness, and the role of health visitors is almost entirely conceived in preventive terms.

Increasingly it is being argued that prospects for prevention and treatment would be enhanced by a closer collaboration between these workers, and the concept of the 'primary health care team' has evolved. Although there has been a steady build-up of partnership practices of general practitioners since the National Health Service began in 1948, the idea of other collaborators has grown most noticeably since the mid 1960s and the General Practice Charter. This Charter was produced by the Minister of Health, the British Medical Association and the Royal College of General Practitioners in 1965–6. It resulted in financial inducements for GPs to work in group practices of three or more partners and offered 70 per cent reimbursement of salaries for employed staff. The attachment of nurses, midwives and health visitors was also encouraged (Pritchard, 1981). In 1968, the Seebohm Report (1968) also recommended that social workers be attached to general practices. The GP is therefore seen to be the lynchpin of the primary care team (Marsh and Meacher, 1979; Pritchard, 1981; Sheppard, 1983). The six main functions of the team are health maintenance, illness prevention, diagnosis and treatment, rehabilitation, care, and certification (Pritchard, 1981).

Collaboration of this sort has indeed materialised over the last twenty-five years. Although a considerable number of single-handed GPs remain, and many small partnerships, many group practices now have four GPs, at least one health visitor and community nurse, and sometimes a practice nurse and a midwife. They will also have a receptionist, and possibly a medical secretary, a practice manager and an administrator (Pritchard, 1981). The community nurse works primarily with the elderly and chronically sick clients of the practice in their own homes, and the practice nurse with minor injuries, immunisations, antenatal checks, urine tests and the like in the surgery. The health visitor has the most obviously preventive role. She is a regular visitor of young children and elderly people, and her visits are not initiated primarily in response to medical symptoms. She acts as educator, counsellor, caring agent, front-line social worker and provider of resources, and is the ears and eyes of the primary health care team in the community (Pritchard, 1981). As she owes her origins to the women sanitary inspectors of 1918 who were attempting to lower the very high infant mortality rate which existed at that time, and although now supposed to care for the whole community, two-thirds of her visits will be to the homes of children under five years old (Pritchard, 1981).

Social work attachments to general practices have increased so that more than 50 per cent of boroughs now have at least one scheme in operation (Clare and Corney, 1982, p. 151). As so many of the complaints presented to the GP have an underlying social or emotional problem (Clare, 1982), many doctors have also looked for assistance in offering counselling. Toynbee (1983) reports that 120 counsellors have been placed in GP surgeries around the country through the voluntary Marriage Guidance Council, mainly dealing with marital and sexual problems. In one county, three practices have been able to secure funds to recruit counsellors by reclaiming 70 per cent of their wages from the Family Practitioners Committee (Graham, 1983). This was made possible by a liberal interpretation of the regulations for reclaiming wages for secretaries, receptionists and clerks. In line with the recommendations of the Trethowan Report (DHSS, 1977) there has also been an increasing number of visiting schemes between clinical psychologists and general practitioners (Jerrom et al., 1983). This does not necessarily require specialist primary care psychology posts, but can be achieved by psychologists based in hospitals visiting surgeries and health centres on a sessional basis (Jerrom et al., 1983).

Psychiatrists too are beginning to work in primary care settings, a trend which has developed silently, on the initiative of individual GPs or psychiatrists rather than following the recommendations of any central organising body (Strathdee and Williams, 1984). A surprisingly large number of psychiatrists, as many as one in five of those sent questionnaires by Strathdee and Williams (1984), reported that they spent some of their working week in GP settings, usually health centres. Most had begun to do so since 1972, and became involved in seeing patients themselves, shifting some of their out-patient service to the primary care setting and taking new patients directly from the GP's referral. Others, however, preferred to offer advice on specific cases and leave the GP to manage them, or in some cases to provide training for the GP in psychiatric skills such as interviewing.

In fact, there seems to be considerable enthusiasm for this kind of collaboration. Strathdee and Williams (1984) report that psychiatrists felt it enabled them to increase their knowledge of the range of illness seen by GPs, to see patients at an earlier stage of difficulty, that it could reduce admissions to hospital, and help GPs to learn management skills for psychiatric problems. In fact, in long-standing schemes, the psychiatrist was sometimes able, after a period of time, to withdraw from a direct role with the practice, but maintain his support for the GP in a supervisory and training capacity. It was also claimed that the scheme was usually operated in addition to the psychiatrist's normal workload, rather than at the expense of other duties.

Cooper and his colleagues (1982) have compared the outcome for clients of a general practice team which had a social worker attached with clients with broadly similar characteristics from practices which did not. Both of the chosen samples had chronic neurotic illnesses. Patients in the former group had fewer clinical symptoms when followed up, more had been taken off psychotropic drugs, and fewer were judged to need continued medical care and supervision. They also showed a greater improvement over the study period (one year) in major areas of social functioning: material conditions, social management and social role satisfaction (Cooper *et al.*, 1982). It may be that the facility to offer social work support as well as medical care will prove to be an effective means of preventing relapse and chronicity among patients with persisting psychiatric problems. Corney (1982) also showed that the use of social workers in a primary health care team was effective in preventing some acute episodes of depression from becoming chronic illnesses. However, results were restricted to one group; women who had been depressed for some time and who had a poor relationship with their spouse or boyfriend found social work support and practical assistance more valuable than other types of intervention such as counselling.

It would seem that a usable framework for preventive mental health work already exists within the British primary care services. Currently, however, the dominant model within the National Health Service is one of illness repair rather than health promotion. Prevention is an implicit, rather than an explicit function of most primary care roles. Few workers would have any clear notion what to do about it if they were more clearly instructed to give greater weight to prevention, or might argue that their day-to-day work can already be seen as largely preventive. However, the Royal College of General Practitioners has been the first of the professional advisory bodies to produce specific suggestions as to how the general practitioner may go about preventing psychiatric disorder among his patients (Royal College of General Practitioners, 1981a; 1981b; 1981c; 1982). The report of the working party on the 'Prevention of Psychiatric Disorders in General Practice' was based on a psychosocial model of mental illness, and focused on problems associated with transitions at four life stages: childhood, adolescence, young adulthood and old age. It suggested how transitions could be made less distressing by offering anticipatory guidance (such as psychological and educational preparation for childbirth, retirement, or surgery); supportive intervention (for example, advice or counselling for a patient going through divorce or who had recently been bereaved); early treatment of pathological reactions; and referral to other supportive agencies (health visitors, self-help groups, social workers). Specific recommendations for work with the elderly, for instance, included anticipatory guidance for changes in residence; encouraging planning and developing good accommodation *before* moving is likely to be dangerous; treating and monitoring the welfare of old people at home; and being cautiously sparing in the use of psychotropic drugs. These recommendations are almost certainly not, at present, widely followed, but the College can be seen to be encouraging preventive practices and trying to create a climate of positive opinion. It is to be hoped that more such thoughtful reports and specific suggestions will be forthcoming from other professional advisory bodies whose members have an implicit role to play in prevention.

(iii) Crisis intervention teams

Crisis intervention has emerged as a method for reducing the numbers of patients needing mental hospital admission throughout Europe and the United States. Cooper (1979) conducted a survey of fifteen crisis units in eight European countries. A multidisciplinary team of physician, nurse and social worker or clinical psychologist is the most common working unit which goes out at short notice to visit people in the community who are in an acute state of distress. The aim has been to respond rapidly and be able to 'stay with the

crisis' (Bouras and Tufnell, 1983). A team in South London explain
how they attempt to marshall support from the family, neighbours
and friends, and any relevant available services such as meals-on-
wheels. The approach is active and positive, aimed at the solution
of problems. Blame is avoided, and the seeking of help seen as a
positive coping response rather than a weakness. But from the outset
it is made clear that the help is short-term and will terminate at a
given point (Bouras and Tufnell, 1983).

A variety of different management techniques can be used by
the helper, ranging from a psychoanalytic approach, through family
therapy, to behaviour therapy and drug use. Some of these involve
a traditional medical role for the helper in which only helper and
client fully participate, but a family-centred approach is favoured by
many (Ratna, 1978). As Ratna describes it, the helper still takes
control of the situation, but suggests that the family is seen together.
Tension is reduced by active support and specific advice, and shared
roles are negotiated towards resolving the crisis. The aim is to make
long-term patient therapy available in case of need, but reduce
anxiety in the home situation so that family members are able to cope
and admission to hospital is avoided. Sometimes, Ratna suggests,
behaviour therapy with the family can be most useful, especially in
situations where their response to difficult behaviour in the client is
inappropriate, perhaps being overcritical of undesired behaviour and
unresponsive to desired behaviour. Positive responses can be encouraged instead, whereby desired behaviour is rewarded and undesired
ignored (Ratna, 1978).

Much of the writing about crisis theory, including the formulations
of Caplan (1964) on crisis intervention, portrays the ideal client as
someone who was hitherto well-adjusted and leading a normal life
in the community but is in an acute state of distress following a
sudden and severe event such as unexpected loss of employment,
bereavement, or breakdown of a key relationship. Assistance at this
critical time to foster good ways of coping was seen as potentially
preventive of consequential psychiatric disorder and protective
against future difficulties in the sense of augmenting the client's
repertoire of coping skills. However, it is clear that the way these
services operate in practice means that the clients are more often
than not people who have a long-standing history of psychiatric
illness who are referred as emergencies with symptoms of a new
acute episode of severe disorder. Bouras and Tufnell (1983) note

that two-thirds of those in their crisis intervention therapy had a previous psychiatric history, involving in-patient treatment. They were referred to the crisis intervention team with a further acute episode, often after losing contact with follow-up services or discontinuing their medication. Cooper (1979) also found that all too often, the units he visited found themselves dealing with the same clients repeatedly. He found little evidence to suggest that the original optimism about prevention and growth through experience had been justified.

Nevertheless, if clients with a psychiatric history and their family and friends can be helped to cope with their difficulties and control the psychiatric symptoms sufficiently to enable the client to maintain his role in the community, then the cycle of recurrent hospitalisation may be broken and future relapse prevented. Indeed, Bouras and Tufnell (1983) reported that they believe that to have been a major benefit of their crisis intervention scheme, that is, the prevention of recurrent morbidity, and that they intended to establish a special community-based rehabilitation team for those clients known to be at high risk for readmission.

There is some evidence that the services have succeeded in reducing mental hospital admissions. Ratna (1978) compared admission rates to a hospital in an area utilising crisis intervention with those to a hospital in a neighbouring area operating traditional hospital psychiatry. He showed that both compulsory admissions and first admissions were lower in the former. Cooper (1979) reported that three of the units he visited were in the process of producing data that seemed likely to show that the setting up of a crisis unit had produced a considerable fall in mental hospital admissions from a defined population over a specified period of time. A possible explanation, of course, is that admissions were simply refused in the area with the crisis service. It is by no means clear that non-admission means that psychiatric disorder has been prevented, and it could just as easily be argued that psychiatric disorder may have been increased. Certainly there has been some evidence that; unless families are well supported by the new service, the mental health of close relatives can be worsened (Sainsbury, 1973).

Considering the expense of crisis and emergency services, remarkably little effort seems to have been given to evaluation; no full-time staff were engaged in evaluative research in any of the fifteen centres visited by Cooper. There is a need, too, for clarity about the aims of these services and about whether, now that the chances of patients being kept in hospital for very long periods becomes negligible, it should necessarily be assumed that admission as such is something to be avoided at all costs. It may be, for instance, that only for certain groups is this assumption correct. For the elderly admission to hospital in itself is often associated with a decline in health and an increased rate of mortality (as noted in earlier paragraphs), and a policy which provides a continuing domiciliary care to enable the elderly to remain in their home setting may well be particularly important in a preventive sense.

Conclusions

Earlier chapters have attempted to set up a theoretical model against which preventive efforts might be assessed. Causal models of depression and schizophrenia have revealed a number of antecedent factors. Theories to explain how the antecedent factors exert their pathogenic effect have been considered and these have pointed to several possible mediating processes and moderating factors which might be open to influence. There is now reasonably convincing evidence that coping skills and social support can have a moderating effect, and self-esteem and helplessness have been put forward as possible mediating processes in the development of depression. And many of the preventive projects described appear to have been effective in these terms. What is almost entirely missing, however, from efforts directed at young children and their families is any evidence that the changes they have produced will affect the chances of those children succumbing to psychiatric disorder in adulthood. And rarely does an investigator suggest how a reduction in disturbed classroom behaviour, say, will have a long-term preventive benefit, or what it is hoped will be prevented once the child is no longer in any classroom. Future longer-term enquiries may begin to answer such questions.

A general impression obtained from this review is that prevention in the field of mental health has primarily concerned itself with an unspecified range of adjustment problems – school maladjustment and truancy, school failure, adolescent delinquency, childhood fears, anxiety associated with medical procedures, the stress of being a single parent, unemployed, carer of a handicapped child or being newly divorced. These problems are considered as a justifiable focus for preventive mental health projects, irrespective of their greater or lesser relevance to the aetiology of psychiatric illness in individual cases. The fact that such variables have been found to be implicated in some way in psychiatric disorder, and in any case are associated with social disadvantage or psychological distress, is seen to warrant a general population approach to their prevention.

Despite the limited theoretical exploration of their preventive practices by most investigators, several of the intervention programmes described in this chapter nevertheless merit serious consideration, as they show promising results in terms of likely long-term preventive benefits. But an issue which recurs as crucial is the identification of those at risk. Those school-based projects which have been specifically directed at a group already showing signs of emerging psychiatric and educational difficulties seem most helpful. Family-centred projects which seem most promising are those which work with families whose multiple psychosocial problems are already becoming manifest in terms of maternal depression and child behaviour problems. Event-centred programmes which hold the most potential are those which use information about people most vulnerable to certain kinds of events to decide which people will be offered the help, and what form the help will take. Programmes aiming to prevent treated psychiatric patients from having recurrent episodes of disorders are also of greatest value to those whose home circumstances put them at particularly high risk of relapse. Each of the high-risk approaches described offer considerable promise for future preventive efforts.

However, this focus on risk status, and the inevitable presence of some psychiatric symptoms in high-risk subjects, raises the difficult issue of whether or not the improvements found can be defined as *prevention*.

Problems of defining benefits of interventions as preventive

It is abundantly clear that no single aetiological factor is sufficient of itself to bring about psychiatric disorder. Both parents may have schizophrenia, or both parents may tragically die leaving their young child's future to be determined by the local authority, or a person may be terribly physically scarred in an industrial accident – but that individual will not necessarily develop a major psychiatric disorder. Only a combination of factors will transform a raised risk into an almost certainty. If only one risk factor is present, such as the immi-

nent occurrence of an event which would to most people be judged
to pose a marked long-term threat, such as being taken into hospital
for a mastectomy operation, the benefits of a preventive counselling
programme would not, in fact, be preventing psychiatric disorder in
most of the women. Other circumstances in the lives of many of the
women would have made a psychiatric outcome unlikely whether or
not they received preventive counselling. Although anxiety about the
pain involved in surgical procedures and physical recovery after the
operation seems almost certain to be modified by anticipatory guidance or counselling support after the event, only for a much smaller
number is it possible that more serious psychiatric sequelae will have
been averted. Only longitudinal prospective studies of women going
through this event can help to specify the factors which would enable
the identification of additional risk factors by which the most vulnerable women could be identified.

Parkes and Raphael have both mounted preventive programmes
for a narrowly defined high-risk group. They used an outcome
measure of benefit to psychological adjustment some twenty months
or so after bereavement. Given that the risk factors were meaningful,
however, it seems almost inevitable that *some* depression would follow
the event before the benefits of counselling would be measurable.
An ambivalent marriage, an unsupportive family, the unexpectedness
of the death are not changed by counselling after the event. Instead,
the counselling aims to help the individual work through his grief,
come to terms with his loss, and reassess his future. Immediately
after the event, and before much counselling support could be
provided, the high-risk group would be very likely to show symptoms
of depression. An assessment of the benefit of the intervention would
need to follow the counselling, at which time, counselled and uncoun-
selled high-risk individuals should show a difference in current symptomatology. But quite probably the two groups will *not* have shown
differences at the time of their loss. This seems to be what happened
not only to Parkes's and Raphael's bereaved subjects, but also to the
unselected sample of mastectomy patients counselled in Maguire's
study. However, while the former investigators extol the preventive
benefits of the method, Maguire considered it to be a failure, because
it did not stop people getting depressed, only shortened the duration
of the depression.

This is perhaps the logical consequence of utilising a disease
model of prevention. An approach which awaits sufficient information

on risk such that an intervention can be justified as likely to avert disorder that could be expected to occur without the programme will often find the target group to already have at least the first symptoms of the disorder. But this does not necessarily mean that the intervention should be considered treatment rather than prevention. The crux of the question in these examples centres on the definition of mental illness. Grief which follows mastectomy or bereavement is normal. In most instances, only if it persists over a longer period of time than normal can it be definable as a mental illness. A consideration of prevention necessitates that a high threshold for the definition of disorder be used (as described in chapter 2). Otherwise all depression could be regarded as mental disorder, which would encourage primary carers to treat it, and discourage volunteers or other non-medical carers from involving themselves. The burden on medical services would be intolerable. If Maguire had defined only severe and protracted depression as mental disorder, as it is suggested he should have done, then, like Parkes and Raphael, he would have concluded that his counselling programme for mastectomy patients was highly successful in preventing mental disorder.

By focusing on a risk group who are experiencing some symptoms of psychiatric disorder, but are not yet mentally ill, there are many tangible and professionally appealing implications for primary care workers. Much could be done to enhance their effectiveness given the increasing liaison between different professional groups both in America and the UK, and their apparent interest in this side of their work. Innovative practices with preventive potential are gradually emerging on an *ad hoc* basis but as yet few have clearly specified preventive goals or evaluative information on their effectiveness. Experimental studies are revealing many hopeful methods which could be taken up within existing services. The practical implications of the prevention research will be discussed in the concluding chapter.

10
The way forward

'Where new knowledge and understanding will take us is not predictable. It is hard to accept the fact that the more you know, the more you need to know and that it is an endless process that does not end in a utopia. There will always be problems. This is the consequence of all new knowledge just as it should be part of the perceived reality of all those who create settings today and dream of future societies.' (Sarason, 1972, p. 284)

From theory to practice: some problems

(i) Evidence of benefit

The problems involved in developing, testing and implementing new ideas have perhaps never been better illustrated than in the history to date of preventive psychiatry. In the study of the origins of major psychiatric illness the long-standing divide between psychology and biology has only begun to narrow over the last twenty-five years, while new conflicts within each discipline continue to open up. Do social factors like family relationships only affect the course of schizophrenia, or do they also contribute to onset? Are social relationships protective against depression, or is the capacity to make good relationships indicative of a personality type that also tends to be resilient to depression? Are the origins of schizophrenia rooted in biochemical anomalies of the brain, or is there a physiological difference in the respective adequacy of the two brain hemisphere? And the conflicts have never merely been academic issues. One approach or another, and consequently, its proponents, is seen to be 'hard' and scientific or well-intentioned but 'soft'. Their respective critics often show more than a little emotional commitment to their viewpoint.

In translating aetiological theories into credible preventive proposals and testing these methods in experimental intervention programmes, progress has been markedly difficult. Although many early obstacles such as the problems of reliably measuring the existence of psychiatric disorder, changes in psychiatric state, and developing tools to assess social environments have to a considerable extent been overcome, sophisticated intervention programmes which fully utilise available knowledge and tools in their design and evaluation are hard to find. Part of the problem may be that most programmes have not been set up by the same groups of people who have worked on the development of the theory, but by practitioners who may have very different priorities and interests. The work on expressed emotion and its effects on the course of schizophrenia is a rare example of a continuity of work by the same group of investigators, and perhaps for this reason is some of the best available information on prevention.

Almost certainly, however, the complexity of current aetiological models accounts for a good deal of the poor research. Consider the model for prevention described in chapter 3. Not only are the factors which precede the development of most psychiatric disorder multiple, but individually each is invariably relatively innocuous. It is the interaction or summation of a variety of factors that is critical. This means that an intervention which modified any one antecedent factor but left others unchanged would stand little chance of having a measurable impact on outcome. However, the effects of the intervention could be assessed more reliably if a good deal was known about other contributing factors. Consider, for instance, a programme aiming to improve the social support of a sample of people thought to be vulnerable to depression because they were single parents with severe financial problems and living isolated lives. It would be helpful to know whether their own childhood had equipped them with good coping skills and positive self-esteem, whether they currently showed helpless attitudes to life or were low in self-esteem, whether they had any work outside the home, whether they had any other major concurrent stresses, and whether there was any family history of psychiatric disorder, as well as a full picture of their existing social relationships and what actual support these relationships were providing. With this information, rate of psychiatric disorder could be studied according to the characteristics of each person on other vulnerability factors, to see whether the intervention was of more help to some people than to others. If, for instance, only a small group seemed to benefit, but these were people with low self-esteem and several current stresses, then it could be concluded that only this group needed this kind of intervention, rather than because the effect of the intervention was very small on the group as a whole, that it was therefore not beneficial. Furthermore, if a full picture of the sample were available before and after the intervention, other possible explanations for any apparent improvements could be sought – perhaps a day nursery opened locally to enable some parents to take up part-time work.

Apart from the wide range of information needed, there is also the difficulty of the time periods involved. If the protective effect of social support can only really be tested in a crisis, the researcher may need to wait a number of years and chart all severe events and difficulties over that period in order to evaluate the intervention. With programmes aiming to modify vulnerability factors at an earlier point in the chain, such as parenting, the time period needed before benefit could be established in terms of reduced risk to adult depression, say, would be substantial. And a great many other factors would need to be monitored in the interval.

As the previous chapter has shown, many investigators have aimed instead to evaluate intervention in terms of intermediate factors. If an improved mother-child relationship can be proved to result from an intervention programme, and is reflected in the child's general adjustment and self-esteem, this is often the best evidence on preventive effectiveness that the researcher can hope for.

(ii) Desire to act

These are some of the very real methodological difficulties involved in establishing the preventive benefits of certain courses of action. However, the very strong commitment of many investigators to find generally applicable solutions has sometimes led them to unrealistic expectations of intervention and an over-readiness to assume that these have in fact been met, or at least to a readiness to recommend action without strong evaluative evidence to support it. For instance, Rickel and her colleagues (1984) describe some of the problems in demonstrating the long-term benefits of pre-school intervention programmes, but nevertheless advocate the routine implementation of early intervention in primary schools. They suggest that pre-school and primary grade teachers should administer brief screening devices to their new pupils each autumn and implement special programmes for problem children. In the same book, Durlak and Jason review programmes of affective education for school-aged children and adolescents. These programmes centre on the development of under-standing of oneself and others, interpersonal problem-solving training and general intrapersonal and interpersonal skills considered to be important in promoting psychological growth and social devel-opment. They conclude that 'research data have yet to clearly estab-lish the preventive value of various affective education programmes' but, on the following page, that 'the primary prevention value of affective education cannot be underestimated' (p. 109). The latter conclusion seems to be based on the availability of the programme to large populations, its efficient and relatively inexpensive method of delivery, and its personal and political acceptability. The fact that the programme has not been shown to be effective in producing significant, desirable outcomes or to have no undesirable side-effects is no deterrent to recommending its implementation.

On the other hand, there are some programmes which have been shown to be beneficial but which are not inexpensive or politically acceptable, and it may well be that these latter features are in fact more significant in determining the direction of practice. In many preparation programmes for children undergoing stressful medical procedures, investigators have worked with nurses who have no administrative power to continue the programme once the research is complete. These programmes may show that a home visit by the nurse is more effective in reducing the child's anxiety and that of his parents, and the child's behavioural adjustment to hospitalisation and medical procedures, than in-hospital preparation. But, as Peterson and Brownlee-Duffeck (1984) ask, how useful is this if most hospitals currently cannot offer preparation for children conveniently located in a ward next to the nursing station?

(iii) Adequacy of resources

Clearly, the successful implementation of a preventive programme will depend not only on its known effectiveness in experimental trials, but also on its personal and political acceptability, the possibility of finding efficient methods of service delivery, and its cost. However, this might suggest that given sufficient resources and political will,

as many people as might be needed can be trained to provide the
services necessary to meet a particular problem. In fact, history shows
that even with the greatest commitment to positive changes, the
people involved in the creation of new programmes frequently fail
to consider the reality of the limitation of resources and that they
may not be adequate to render the quantity or quality of service to
those eligible for it (Sarason, 1972). When this happens, the problem
of resources markedly increases as the programme becomes functional and becomes one of its major complaints. This seems to be
what happened in the establishment of the community mental health
centre programme in the United States. President Kennedy's special
message in 1963 announcing this programme promised comprehensive facilities for all aspects of mental health care, located in the
patient's own community. Prevention as well as treatment would
be a major activity of the centres. He recommended that federal
government provide between half and three-quarters of the funds
for their construction, and up to 75 per cent of their staffing costs,
in the early months. An expansion of clinical, laboratory and field
research in mental illness was also recommended, and a sharp
increase in all key professional and auxiliary practitioners. As Sarason
(1972, p. 104) observes, 'rarely in a situation of recognised scarcity
was so much promised to so many'. As Leighton (1982) has since
described, the managers of community mental health centres soon
realised the impossibility of achieving their goals, particularly in
regard to servicing the very extensive potential client group for whom
they were charged with promoting mental health. Of course their
problems were more complicated than a straightforward failure to
consider resources, but Leighton's descriptions of the fate of many
community mental health centre programmes show that they have
tended to follow the disappointing path described by Sarason. Staff
lost their shared sense of mission, became caught up in all kinds of
strife, turnover began to escalate. Disillusionment set in and the work
became routine. The setting then takes on some of the characteristics
of practices it was intended to replace.

(iv) Threat to existing resources and practices

However, while it might seem that a programme which was demonstrably effective, acceptable and affordable should pass smoothly into formal policy and practice, history again shows that more often than not it will still fail when implemented. Sarason (1972) describes his involvement in the setting up of numerous new programmes; from new schools to psychiatric rehabilitation centres and innovative treatment services, and their alarming propensity to fail. 'Time and again I have observed the creation of settings (usually in the human services area) with whose basic values and aims it would be hard to disagree, only to see over time how optimism is replaced by pessimism, consensus by polarisation, and passionate concern for values by a desire to exist' (p. 20). One of the sources of this disastrous cycle lies, firstly, in the implications of the new service for the way existing resources must be redistributed. Furthermore, the new programme will inevitably be championed as ideologically superior to previous modes of operation and in this sense is an indictment of the ways in which traditional agencies attempted to meet the needs they were intending to serve. This ideology and competition for resources virtually ensures some conflict between existing programmes and the new one. For instance, Sarason quotes extensively from a report of the setting up of a residential youth centre in New Haven as part of a 'War on Poverty' programme (described more fully in Goldenberg, 1971). It aimed to help disadvantaged young people settle into independent accommodation and the world of work. Inevitably the proposals for the project were seen as a criticism of existing work and poverty programmes and related agencies. The proposal for funding was immediately rejected by the office responsible for the existing programmes.

Secondly, existing services have long-established operational procedures, professionals are trained to think and work in particular ways, and professional boundaries are commonly understood and observed. A new programme which requires changes to firmly held traditions will run into all kinds of practical problems. By way of example, Sarason summarises the fate of an innovative management programme for patients with chronic schizophrenia, from a detailed report by Colarelli and Siegel (1966). One hospital ward, 'Ward H', was restructured and developed according to guiding principles derived from a set of conceptions about aetiological factors in schizophrenia. A pilot study had produced promising results, and the project was received warmly and enthusiastically by staff in the rest of the hospital. But within a year of becoming a reality a series of crises had arisen. Nursing aides had had anxieties about their newfound authority, other supporting professional staff withdrew their commitment, and the supervising nurse resigned because the methods were too discrepant with her background and training. There was concern from the hospital administration about the low level of contact between physician and patients, and difficulties in filling staff vacancies through the lengthy established procedures. Even painting the walls of the ward by aides and patients caused conflicts with the painters in the maintenance section of the hospital.

From all available evidence, the project was very successful. Their patients had often been assumed not to be amenable to treatment, but discharge rates from Ward H were as high as for the rest of the hospital, and readmission was dramatically lower. The personnel cost was equivalent to that of the least expensive ward in the hospital. But within four years, the project ceased. It could not be absorbed into the existing setting.

(v) Perceived boundaries of psychiatry

It seems that the problems which have been encountered in obtaining evaluative information from experimental projects may well be dwarfed by the awesome difficulties involved in the general implementation of the programmes. A wide range of anxieties continue to be raised about the introduction of preventive practices by practitioners within existing services. In formulating policies for the development of community psychiatric care in Britain, for instance, it has been recognised that the role of the psychiatrist will be wider, and that he or she will be involved in work with a broader range of clients (Freeman, 1983). This is perceived by many as posing a real threat to the quality of care for severely and chronically mentally ill people in that resources might be diverted from this already overstretched area of work (e.g. Richman and Barry, 1985). This concern is not surprising given some of the disturbing accounts of the aftermath of deinstitutionalisation in some American cities where many chronic psychotic patients have been decanted into nursing homes, boarding homes, flop houses and the street (Brown, P., 1985). Richman and Barry argue that psychiatry should not expand its boundaries to encompass whole communities, but should become more like other medical specialities, and stick more clearly to the defined disease states, with definite guidelines about which patients they serve, for which mental and bodily functions, and with which goals.

This line of argument appears to assume that only those people currently treated by psychiatrists have a 'real' mental illness and that those who have not hitherto tended to receive specialist treatment have mild disorders or transient illnesses that will clear up without help in a relatively short space of time. However, as documented in chapter 2, community surveys using reliable diagnostic criteria with a high cut-off point to determine the presence and severity of disorder have revealed a good deal of disorder remaining untreated in the general population which is of equal severity and duration to that treated by psychiatrists (Brown *et al.*, 1985). The depressed women identified by Brown and his colleagues were more likely to have seen a psychiatrist if they also showed signs of personality disturbance and acting out behaviour, suggesting that the mode of expression of symptoms is at least as important as their presence in determining who receives treatment. Tennant and his colleagues (1981) found that more than half the depressive episodes detected in the community did remit within four months, and Brown and his colleagues found two-thirds cleared up within thirty-nine weeks. However, this leaves a substantial number of illnesses which persist. While this may be a relatively small proportion of those who become cases in any year, the numbers obviously accumulate such that at any one time, half the depressed women in the community will have a chronic condition (Brown *et al.*, 1985; Surtees *et al.*, 1983). Should the common cold tend to become chronic in a proportion of cases, no doubt considerably more effort would be devoted to its prevention. The clear-up rate for depression is particularly low amongst the poor and elderly (Murphy, 1983).

However, this must mean that improved systems in primary care for detecting early signs of psychiatric disorder will considerably increase the potential client group of mental health services. It also means that if effective preventive services were offered, the effects would not be accurately measurable in terms of a reduction of cases presenting for psychiatric care. It is quite possible that a preventive programme in general practice could be effective in preventing considerable psychiatric morbidity, but have almost no effect on the numbers of patients treated by psychiatrists. Furthermore, greater links between psychiatry and general practice could drain the specialist service of senior and talented staff. A community psychiatric nurse might be able to counsel a large number of patients in general practice, help them to deal more effectively with their problems, catch early signs of psychiatric disorder, and avert the need for referral to hospital. But as he or she is likely to be of senior nurse status, a substantial number of hospital referrals might need to be avoided before it proved to be less costly (in financial terms) to do this than to await the referral of the patient to the hospital.

(vi) Motivation of practitioners

A final problem in the implementation of preventive practices on a general population scale concerns the motivation of practitioners. How can the family physician, say, whose main concern is often in treating presenting symptoms, be motivated to take an interest in prevention? The introduction of financial inducements has success-fully increased routine immunisations. The family practitioner committee provides 70 per cent of the wages of practice nurses if the practice operates as recommended in the 1966 Charter. However, this kind of approach seems unlikely to be appropriate for preventive counselling.

That general practitioners do not, by and large, currently practice as much preventive medicine as they might seems to be illustrated by their record in preventing two common physical disorders, type 2 diabetes and uncomplicated hypertension. A review in the *Lancet* (1984) describes results from a number of comparative studies. One compared the management of diabetic people randomly allocated to continued care at a hospital diabetic clinic or to the care of their general practitioner. Over the five-year follow-up, only 14 per cent of the latter group were reviewed at least once a year, compared to 100 per cent of the hospital group, and three times as many had died! Another study of patients admitted to hospital in a ketoacidotic coma found over half (fifteen of twenty-seven) with undiagnosed diabetes, and despite a total of forty-one visits to their family doctors, twelve of the fifteen had not had their urine tested.

Similarly damning evidence exists in screening for hypertension. Several studies have documented the failure of family doctors to check the blood pressure of patients, even when they have been

started on anti-hyptertensive drugs and their risk status is therefore
clear. Only one out of three men over the age of twenty have been
found to have had their blood pressure recorded at any time during
the previous ten years (see the *Lancet*, 1984). The evidence seems
to reflect a general unstated policy of waiting for the customer to
initiate every demand and then to practise a system of illness repair.
Perhaps this is to some extent a reflection of the emphasis in the
training of doctors, or the motivation of people to become doctors,
or the satisfaction gained from helping ill people to get well compared
to the invisibility of illness that has been prevented.

Daunting theoretical and operational problems will therefore have
to be overcome in implementing preventive proposals.

From theory to practice: towards what kind of optimum practice does the research evidence point?

Given that there will be many potential obstacles to successful intervention which must be borne in mind, what programmes should we
be striving to develop? What conclusions can be drawn from this
review about the most promising ways forward?

First and foremost, a good start in life has fundamental importance
in laying the foundations for resilience or vulnerability to childhood
and adult psychiatric disturbance. Advantage comes not from material
resources as such, but from the quality of the child's experience of
being parented – from the security of knowing that one or more of
his primary caretakers are seriously concerned about his welfare and
from their provision of guidance on how he is expected to conduct
himself. Of course, this is hardly a surprising conclusion; it is a
conclusion which has been reached by psychologists and psychiatrists
time and again over the last half-century and seems self-evident to
most lay persons. Yet many of our social policies do not seem to give
the priority to policies affecting family life which might be expected.

For parents to fulfil their role as well as possible, they need to
derive pleasure, satisfaction and a sense of value from attempting to
do so. They need to live in homes which provide defensible play
space for children, and which maximise opportunities for social
contacts with other families. They need sufficient child benefit to
free them from poverty-line income, which would also help to
demonstrate the value which society places on parenting. Mothers
need to be able to find employment outside the home if they wish,

which means that there need to be more opportunities for job sharing, flexible work hours, and part-time work. Such flexible employment practices would also enable partners to share the parenting role, and if they were sufficiently widespread, may increase the opportunities for other unemployed groups. And perhaps a tax allowance should be considered to make working an economic feasibility if supplementary child care arrangements need to be purchased.

Parents without the education, experience, material resources and emotional support to enable them to effectively and enjoyably fulfil their parenting role need to be provided with some of these resources. Young women need to be prepared for the enormously difficult task of motherhood every bit as thoughtfully as they are prepared for a healthy birth. When they arrive home with their new baby they need mother and baby groups within the neighbourhood where they can find friends with children of the same age and from whom they can seek advice and support on child management problems. As well as the existing opportunities to discuss their child's health and development with their local health visitor, they need other sources of easily intelligible advice and information on general child management: cartoon leaflets on what to do about the baby's night-time waking perhaps, as provided by health visitors in the Child Development Programme described in the last chapter; lunchtime television programmes which dramatise common child management problems and possible solutions, perhaps; or telephone advice services of the same nature.

For parents with persisting difficulties with their children, intense health visiting support might be considered, or referral to voluntary mum-to-mum befriending services where they exist. These may to some extent replace the function which until recently was served by members of the extended family. The aim of these efforts should be to work with the mother to improve her capacity to guide and support her child and derive a sense of self-esteem and self-efficacy from her success. Approaches which focus on the child alone at this stage would serve to reinforce the parents' dependency on professionals and their view of themselves as ineffective in influencing their child's behaviour. Beneficial effects on the child would therefore be likely to be temporary.

When families with pre-school children have had many psycho-social difficulties and parenting problems, and home-based programmes have either not been provided or have not prevented

behavioural or emotional problems in the child, then emerging difficulties can be picked up at school. At this stage, it is less likely that
professional child-centred intervention will undermine parents, as
some responsibility for the child's behavioural and cognitive development will already have been handed over to teachers. And there is
evidence from several school-based intervention programmes that
early-detected conduct disorder can be improved. The methods
which have been found to be successful require a high level of
training and short-term extra curricular sessions for children in their
first two or three years at school, who have been revealed, through
screening procedures, to be showing early signs of conduct disorder.
There are also implications in this research for the training of
teachers. Very little preparation is given to teachers in training on
how to deal with disruptive and difficult children, and more advice
and support for their efforts would seem warranted.

However, although intervention has so far focused primarily on
methods of early treatment of emerging disorder or on the enhancement of problem-solving skills, some of the most recent research
suggests that other kinds of intervention might actually be expected
to be *more* effective in the long term. The evidence suggests that
screening for children whose parenting is particularly neglectful and
making special efforts to find rewarding and enjoyable experiences
for them in school would be preventive of psychiatric disorder to the
extent to which it augmented their ability to take control of and plan
their lives, and reduced feelings of helplessness.

At the age at which many young people unintentionally become
parents, there needs to be more education to encourage them to act
responsibly: perhaps a campaign aimed at adolescent boys and young
men, similar to the 'Men Too' campaign proposed by the Family
Planning Association in England, to take the initiative in contraception; perhaps a campaign for adolescent girls to persuade them to be
more assertive in insisting on it, maybe something akin to the current
'Say No' campaigns against drug abuse. For children reared under
the guardianship of the local authority, the responsibilities of that
authority to act as a good parent should extend beyond some arbitrary
age cut-off point. Support is needed while teenagers establish themselves in satisfactory living circumstances in order to reduce the very
high rate of premarital pregnancies amongst girls raised in care.

A sense of control over the events of one's life also has fundamental
importance to the resilience of adults to a range of psychiatric

disorders, but particularly to depression. Yet many work conditions, housing conditions, and some patterns of institutional care act to minimise people's sense of (and opportunities for) self-determination and as such increase their susceptibility to psychiatric illness. This is often true in care arrangements for elderly, disabled or disturbed people. There are self-evident implications for planners of such institutions, the carers running them, for employers and for town planners.

In adulthood there are a wide range of events and difficulties which may pose sufficient threat to individuals as to considerably raise the possibility that they will develop a psychiatric disorder. A few events, such as marital separation (for the partner who is left alone) have a degree of generalisable threat, that is, most people left by their spouse will perceive the event as posing a marked long-term threat. Many other events, however, will vary much more widely in their interpretation by individuals, according to the circumstances of their lives. Much more longitudinal research is needed on individuals experiencing common worrying and distressing events to reveal factors predictive of psychiatric disorder. There is no generalisable remedy available to help people adapt to events of different kinds; valuable resources, coping skills and support will be dependent on the nature of the event. However, some events are sufficiently common and occur to people in sufficiently accessible environments to provide ready opportunities for experimental preventive programmes: operations, stillbirth, physical disablement and bereavement occur to people in hospitals. Counselling, befriending and stress-management techniques should be evaluated.

Professional psychiatric services for crisis intervention have had most success in terms of preventing the need for acutely disturbed individuals to be admitted to hospital. But to have a genuinely preventive role in terms of reducing the likelihood of relapse, they might more effectively deploy their resources in identifying those discharged psychiatric patients at greatest risk of relapse, and offering intensive domiciliary support programmes to this group. Such programmes would include family therapy programmes for relatives of patients treated for schizophrenia on optimum ways of helping the ex-patient to remain well. They would include preparing the individual for new placements in rehabilitation centres or training schemes, and a careful monitoring of and support in finding good accommodation and daytime occupation.

From theory to practice: some answers

(i) Maximising the pay-off of action

The complex chain of adverse circumstances and events which may culminate in psychiatric disorder can potentially be interrupted at one of several different stages. In general the more advanced the stage, the more accurate can be the identification of risk. Few people who move away from family ties and close friends to take a job in a foreign country will become depressed. But if the person fails to establish new friendships, and in fact finds himself subject to racial harassment and the job to fall far short of expectations, the risk of psychiatric disorder may be greater. If he has problems coping with the job, begins to take days off from work and reports to the company doctor with a variety of mild physical complaints, it would not be surprising to find that he already has a number of psychiatric symptoms. While a preventive programme for all immigrants would not, for the great majority of the recipients, be preventing psychiatric disorder, for those picked up with mild symptoms in doctors' surgeries, the possibility that it could arrest or avert serious disorder, should it be effective, would be much greater. The maximum pay-off of intervention in this scenario would therefore be to screen for the first signs of psychiatric problems in primary health care settings.

A variety of screening questionnaires has been developed. It may even be possible that a handful of questions may be identified which provide a relatively high accuracy in detecting psychiatric problems among patients who consult their physician for physical complaints as long as it is accepted that there will be many false positives (the GHQ is already available in a twelve-item version). These questions may then be incorporated routinely into a doctor's discussions with his or her patients. The early detection and treatment of depression may well lead to a considerable reduction in its duration (Maguire et al., 1980; Johnstone and Goldberg, 1976). It seems likely that referrals to agencies able to help alleviate the client's social difficulties may also be effective in reducing existing psychiatric symptoms and the further development of the disorder. In the above example there may, for instance, be a supportive local community group to whom the general practitioner could refer his patient, and through whom the man could find friendships and social activities.

Of course, the problem of motivation remains. Only a certain proportion of general practitioners are likely to be sufficiently concerned with preventive mental health work to implement such ideas. And others will consider they have more than enough difficulty in providing treatment for the illnesses which cry out for attention without attempting to uncover others. Nevertheless, general practitioners have a good number of regular attenders at the surgery whom they feel unable to help, and they may look favourably on schemes which promise to reduce this group. General practitioners who were interested in such ideas, but not in providing counselling themselves, may be able to strike up profitable links with locally based psychiatrists, psychologists, marriage guidance counsellors or other counsellors who might be offered their own surgeries within the practice. The GP could use the screening techniques and then offer the patient the opportunity to talk to the practice counsellor if psychiatric problems were detected. In his turn the counsellor could have an army of community contacts for further supportive referral if other more specific types of support were needed (befriending groups, mutual aid and the like).

Waiting for a person to seek medical help is not the only effective way of finding those people particularly likely to be showing early signs of psychiatric illness. The high-risk individual will often have a range of social difficulties as well as a life history which predisposes him to develop psychiatric disorder when faced with acute difficulties. Some of the intervention programmes aiming to help high-risk people have shown that it is not a difficult matter to identify their target group. For instance, in his studies of bereaved persons most likely to develop persistent psychiatric disorders, Parkes (1981) found that one of the most useful predictive factors was an intuitive guess by staff nursing the dying patient and meeting his or her relatives as to how well or how badly they were likely to be able to cope with the loss. The befriending service described by Pound and her colleagues (1985) sought referrals from health visitors, general practitioners, social workers and other clients and volunteers. They were asked to refer mothers of young children with problems of depression, isolation and child management. Most, if not all of the referrals turned out to have a life history characterised by the kinds of risk factors which seem so often to be implicated in depression: neglectful parenting, premarital pregnancy, or a lack of a close supportive relationship.

It may turn out to be a similarly straightforward matter to identify those treated psychiatric patients who will be most at risk of relapse when discharged. A simple enquiry into the patient's home circumstances from the patient himself and from any professional with knowledge of such may correlate with actual risk as well as sophisticated, costly and time-consuming research procedures. Or perhaps a rapid readmission after the first discharge would be a valid indication of subsequent risk of relapse. The undoubtedly expensive intensive follow-up support services that have sometimes been recommended, or family therapy programmes, may then be cost-effective, if provided only for a small number of treated patients at greater risk of relapse.

Furthermore, support programmes for people at high risk of developing psychiatric disorder or showing early symptoms of disorder may also be an appropriate early preventive measure for close relatives of the target individual. Those living with a spouse, son or daughter who experiences frequent relapses of schizophrenia may well also experience some psychological benefit of information, advice and practical support in coping with their relatives' disorder. The children whose mother is becoming depressed and seems unable to cope with their needs or organise her home life should benefit in the long term from any improvements in their mother's psychological health brought about by befriending schemes or other support programmes. Indeed, all the evidence points to the appropriateness of directing preventive programmes for young children at their mothers.

It seems to make sense to wait until a sufficiently strong indication of psychiatric risk is apparent before mounting preventive programmes targeted towards people experiencing current adverse circumstances and events rather than offering programmes to an undifferentiated group facing some threatening event. However, there may also be possibilities for the prevention of developmental vulnerability to adversity. Consider, for instance, the links which have been established between early lack of care in the child's parenting, adolescent pregnancy, and vulnerability to adult depression. Preventive efforts might be directed at any or all of three stages. It might be possible to improve the parent-child relationship, perhaps through intensive health visiting support programmes for mothers with parenting problems. It may also be feasible to prevent adolescent pregnancy, perhaps through assertion training or providing opportunities to derive self-esteem and a sense of self-efficacy at school, as well as by providing contraceptive information. Or it might be possible to prevent ineffective coping responses to an unwanted pregnancy, perhaps by offering counselling to all teenagers at their first antenatal visit. However, although there is a considerably raised risk of adult disorder among children experiencing a marked lack of care, it is nevertheless the case that most neglected children will not develop psychiatric problems as adults. The pay-off of intervention in this sequence of adversity may therefore be maximised if screening procedures could identify those teenage girls who were low in self-esteem or a sense of control over their lives. Programmes aiming to improve their self-confidence and sense of mastery which also emphasised avoiding unwanted pregnancy might be the most effective approach. Further research is needed to enable the ready identification of risk indicators such as these.

Finally, a preventive programme that may only reduce the risk of psychiatric disorder among a very small proportion of a target group may be justifiable if it is relatively easy and inexpensive to provide – if, for instance, it simply involves a different way of structuring the environment, perhaps reducing the numbers of class changes for pupils in their first year at secondary school, or training staff caring for elderly residents of institutions to behave in ways which ensure maximum opportunity for self-determination by the residents, rather than encouraging dependent behaviour.

If risk status is to be used as a means of maximising the pay-off of intervention, then research is needed to provide the instruments or key questions which can practicably be used to give a reasonably accurate and easily obtained indication of that risk. Furthermore, much is assumed about the causal significance of many identified indicators of risk, and properly evaluated experimental interventions which use these indicators is one of the most hopeful ways forward for confirming or disproving their causal role.

(ii) Using community resources

The cost of preventive programmes, even if aimed only at a relatively small group of people who have been identified as particularly likely to develop psychiatric symptoms, may still be extremely high if they demand a good deal of professional time. And it has often been assumed that the solution of most mental health problems requires certain kinds of personnel, that these personnel are specialists, and that despite being expensive and in short supply, they can be trained in sufficient number to meet a very wide range of needs (Sarason,

1972). But as Sarason has argued, specialised resources can never be adequate, and decisions must inevitably be made about who should get any given service. A broad range of provision therefore requires innovative solutions involving non-specialists and voluntary help from members of the community.

For instance, the bereavement counselling service provided by St Christopher's Hospice and evaluated by Parkes (1981) used trained volunteer counsellors and was estimated by him to require approximately three days of a social worker's time and three to four hours from a consultant psychiatrist per month. This enabled 400 to 500 families to be screened per year and 100 of these bereaved persons to be given a follow-up counselling service. Given that his research also enabled bereaved people at greatest risk of psychiatric disorder to be identified, it seemed likely that the counselling would reduce consultations with general practitioners and the prescription of minor tranquillisers and sedatives. Parkes concludes that the low cost and proven benefits of this service in terms of reductions in symptoms of anxiety and depression make it reasonable to suggest that it should be more widely available. After a brief training and some months of experience in the service, volunteers were able to become as effective as professionals.

However, it is not advocated that volunteers be used as unpaid professionals or to fulfil roles that would otherwise be filled by professionals. In any case, their most valuable resource for many projects lies in their non-professional role and status. For instance, it has become well-known that many of the most disadvantaged and distressed people in the community do not make use of professional resources intended specifically for them. Families not using health clinics, playgroups and nurseries are often highly alienated people, sometimes lonely, depressed and suspicious. They may even be fearful, of both services and service givers (Eyken, 1982). Eyken describes the lack of a sense of control of these families who are often socially isolated, having problems in child management and also failing to establish more general relationships. When the children reach school age, these are the absentee parents whom no school teacher would see. A befriending service, however, is much more likely to reach this target group. An offer of friendship from someone who is in many ways similar to the referred person can help build up the client's confidence. For many families, it has been suggested that it is also a prerequisite for the subsequent uptake of services (Eyken, 1982).

It is clear from the accounts of those projects in which voluntary helpers provide the main support system that their success, in terms of benefit to clients and degree of commitment of the volunteer, is to a considerable extent influenced by the organisation and management of the project. Volunteers need training and back-up support, to be matched carefully to the clients they befriend, and to derive a sense of achievement or fulfilment from their efforts. And methods of recruiting volunteers will obviously determine who offers to join the scheme. Homestart preferred to discourage those who might not have been able to offer a high level of commitment by their method of advertising for recruits. People unable to devote a full day to training at the outset would not have applied.

Voluntary projects are often able to offer something that the professional cannot. Equally, there are many things the voluntary sector cannot and should not be expected to do. They ought not to replace a statutory function. They differ in more ways than salary and training. But frequently the referrals to voluntary agencies must come from the client list of local social workers, general practitioners and health visitors and there can be an uneasy relationship between the voluntary and statutory service. Homestart, for instance, depends on word-of-mouth recommendations of professional caregivers, and therefore on what the professional considers a suitable case for referral. Inevitably this will vary between professionals, as will their cooperation and enthusiasm. Some social workers, for instance, might perceive the involvement of a volunteer in one of his or her client families as threatening. They might be particularly anxious, too, about the possibility that something might go wrong in some of their more difficult cases for which they will be held responsible (Eyken, 1982). Eyken argues that voluntary and statutory services should not simply operate in partnership but that they should be seen as complementary components of a single service. The voluntary component 'should be both separate from and independent of statutory control' and 'the statutory sector should ensure that this independent function both exists and thrives within the community.' At present, their coexistence is threatened, as the budgets and sometimes the supply of clients to the voluntary service are controlled by the statutory sector. Without giving any clues as to how it might be

achieved, Eyken suggests that new mechanisms be sought to support
the voluntary sector independently of the statutory services.

(iii) Health service implications

What are the implications for the practising psychiatrist or clinical
psychologist of attempting to provide preventive programmes? In line
with Caplan (1964), Gottlieb (1983), and Sarason (1972), it has been
argued here that it is not only inappropriate but impossible for whole
groups of specialist mental health clinicians to take on a front-line
role as direct caregivers of preventive services. But this is not to
advocate for maintenance of the status quo in which prevention is
an assumed function of a variety of professional groups, but not an
explicitly stated aim of any, and a very marginal activity in most as
they attempt first of all to service infinite demands for treatment. Of
all the professional advisory bodies in Britain, only the Royal College
of General Practitioners explicitly states prevention as a key function
of their professional group, and produces guidelines and specific
suggestions as to how the family doctor can improve his preventive
practice (Royal College of General Practitioners, 1981a; 1981b;
1981c; 1982). But surely psychiatry should provide some professional
lead, and be able to supply advice, guidance and support to the
preventive efforts of primary care workers and voluntary groups? The
diverse practices mounted in the name of mental health prevention
are clearly in need of pulling together, of some theoretical base, and
of evaluation of effectiveness. Psychiatrists and psychologists could
perhaps be expected to identify promising approaches to prevention
and encourage existing projects or initiate experimental projects
themselves. Replication of positive effects is one of the ways in which
the spread of good practice might be encouraged. They might help
to ensure that some relevant assessment procedures are incorporated
into new projects from their initiation, from which effectiveness might
be judged. They might provide training and advice to counsellors or
project leaders in their attempts to support distressed and disturbed
people in the community. They might provide back-up support for
the referral of psychiatric difficulties with which project leaders feel
unable to deal. And they might help to establish some interprofessional dialogue with the same purposes for primary care workers.
In short, their role might be as Gottlieb and Caplan suggest, as
consultants, group initiators, trainers and advocates. None of these

activities need seriously distract the clinician from his or her central role of managing illness.

Perhaps the structures within psychiatry for which the implementation of preventive proposals seems most appropriate are the existing services for child guidance and crisis intervention. Much of their work is explicitly aimed at prevention. And given the established problems of finding time or motivation for prevention when preventive work is meant to be undertaken by the same person as the curative work, a case could be made for entrusting professionals in these services with the exclusive responsibility for developing preventive work. There could be prevention specialists and curative specialists, whose roles are defined as differently as those of health visiting nurses and hospital nurses. Furthermore, both child guidance and crisis intervention teams are already staffed by workers from social services and/or psychology as well as psychiatry, and therefore have the framework for interdisciplinary cooperation.

Although child guidance units and crisis intervention teams have preventive aims, discussion in preceding chapters has described the ineffectiveness of these services in preventive terms. Some of the changes which would be needed for more explicitly preventive operations would include a much greater role for staff from child guidance clinics in schools. Child guidance staff could help to set up and run extra-curricular therapy groups for disturbed pupils, and gradually train teaching staff to take over their role. Parent training sessions on the management of behavioural problems in children could also be mounted. Relevant programmes could be started by child guidance staff, and when running, acceptable and effective could be handed over to specially trained teachers. When this was successfully achieved, only a back-up support for teachers, and help in dealing with children the teacher was unable to help, would be needed. The sequence of action would therefore be advocate, group initiator, trainer and consultant.

Preventive child psychologists and other members of the prevention team could also help to instigate community befriending programmes for families with multiple psychosocial problems. They could liaise with local hospitals to try to improve the preparation given to children admitted for lengthy stays in hospital and for distressing surgical procedures. There could be considerably increased cooperation between health visitors and the child guidance team, the latter perhaps offering a supportive back-up facility for health visitors when they encountered particularly severe problems.

Members of crisis intervention teams would become psychiatric relapse preventive specialists. This would extend their role beyond intervention in crisis situations. It would involve the identification of treated patients at greatest risk of relapse and an intense programme of follow-up support to try to change adverse home, work and social circumstances such that relapse was made less likely.

As so much of the psychiatric morbidity in the community is dealt with by the general practitioner and never reaches the psychiatrist, and an even greater number of distressed, high-risk individuals are seen there every day, the psychiatrist's or psychologist's potential importance as consultant is perhaps greatest here. And in fact, as already noted, there has been a rapid growth of liaison or attachment schemes between psychiatrists and general practitioners over the last ten or fifteen years, largely at the initiative of individual practitioners (Strathdee and Williams, 1984). One in five respondents to a survey by Strathdee and Williams (a total of 154 consultant psychiatrists) indicated that they or their junior colleagues spent some time in a general practice setting. And accounts of their experiences are typically enthusiastic. The main benefit of the liaison is seen to be to increase the skills and confidence of the family doctor in detecting and treating both early signs of psychiatric disorder and managing more advanced illnesses, such that fewer referrals to psychiatrists are needed (Williams and Clare, 1981; Mitchell, 1985).

However, the psychiatrist also benefits from working with new colleagues, becoming more aware of the range of disorder seen by general practitioners, learning to make his traditional skills more relevant, and learning more of the social and family backgrounds of clients. Crisis intervention becomes more of a reality and his educational and research role may improve his job satisfaction. For patients who might otherwise need to be seen in out-patient settings there are obvious advantages: less travel, less stigma, greater continuity of care and a greater chance that relatives will be prepared to become involved. Treatment compliance improves and hence deterioration and relapse of psychotic disorders is reduced (see Mitchell, 1985).

Mitchell (1985) describes five different ways in which an attachment scheme might operate, and the relative advantages of each. The arrangement most similar to the approach advocated by Caplan is one in which the psychiatrist does not see any of the GP's patients, but comes to the health centre or surgery for regular group discussions. The group (the GPs and psychiatrist or even the whole primary health care team) can decide for themselves what use they will make of the sessions. The sessions may, for instance, be primarily educational, where screening, case definition, diagnosis or management is discussed. The group may discuss particular patients, or they may be more research-oriented.

Evaluative research has begun on the effectiveness of attachment schemes in reducing hospital admissions and on the extent to which the schemes are flooded by irrelevant referrals. Given that they involve the time of the most senior psychiatrists, their benefit must be measurable in terms of improved quality of service for patients without jeopardising treatment of severe disorders in hospital settings. But beyond their cost efficiency there is the opportunity they also provide for research, for evaluating and supporting local voluntary initiatives, for piloting new screening techniques, for assessing some of the new forms of cognitive therapy for the management of depression, or perhaps for evaluating experimental programmes of anticipatory guidance.

There will also be issues of local and more general concern relevant to prevention on which it is appropriate that the psychiatrist or psychologist should pass comment. Concern has recently been expressed, for instance, on the level of lead in petrol and its effects on the cognitive development of children living in the vicinity of heavy traffic. Some of the research reviewed in earlier chapters has implications for supporting adolescents as they leave local authority residential care, for the management of homes for the elderly, and for the provision of follow-up support for treated psychiatric patients. It may be that Community Health Councils in Britain already provide the forum for the discussion of local plans and policies and in other countries community mental health centres may also facilitate the consideration of local issues.

A concern for the whole person and the whole community underlies the shift in emphasis from treatment in large mental hospitals to care as close as possible to the patient's home. But the training for community psychiatry has hardly begun in this country (Freeman, 1985). Training is still primarily related to diagnosis and drug treatment, and cannot be said to prepare clinicians for many of the activities allied to preventive aspirations. It seems likely that the training of different health care and social workers will need to overlap more than at present, both in content and administration, if greater interprofessional cooperation and understanding is to be achieved.

The evidence that a change in attitude of health care workers can improve their preventive achievements is becoming apparent from the management of many physical disorders in general practice. Even more influential, however, is the organisation and management of a treatment service. The disappointing picture painted in the *Lancet* (1984) of the success of general practitioners in preventing deaths resulting from diabetes and hypertension was counterbalanced by an account of how effective they *can* be. Practitioners who have changed their policy of waiting for the client to initiate every demand and set up mini-clinics for monitoring diabetics or for screening for hypertension have been able to provide as effective a service as specialised hospital clinics. But to manage all the disorders which are currently frequently handled by hospital out-patients departments obviously implies a much increased workload for the general practitioner. This can only be manageable by computer-assisted records and more imaginative work sharing with nurses and receptionists (*Lancet*, 1984). This is the sort of management encouraged by the 1966 Charter, but which GPs are still free to ignore. A variety of suggestions has been put forward to increase the accountability of the general practitioner, including designating him as a medical officer of health reporting both to his family practitioner committee and local registered population on these matters (see the *Lancet*, 1984). Should we not aim to make the guardians of the nation's health more accountable?

A concern for prevention is continuing to permeate the thinking of the general public. Increasingly we question whether our diet is healthy, our environment free from pollutants, our bodies in trim. Psychiatry is also increasingly considering the social and physical environment of its client group. While knowledge of causes and evidence of the effectiveness of intervention is fundamental to advocating preventive practice, changes are nevertheless more likely to be brought about within a general climate of positive popular opinion. Conviction arises slowly, and not necessarily in line with replication of effectiveness. How did the now ubiquitous playgroups for 3–5-year-olds start to proliferate? And ideas and methods that are trusted in other areas are more easily adopted. Family therapy is an established treatment and may be accepted as a potential preventive technique more easily than many novel approaches that do not have a successful track record elsewhere.

The tide is sweeping in prevention's direction. We can be optimistic about the future. We have a good deal of information about risk. We know something about how and why disorder develops. We have some understanding of why some people are resilient.

But we know less about how to intervene to create resilience. And we have a history of failure in attempts to implement preventive practices, even when the method is known to be effective. Enthusiasm and extreme caution are both essential attributes for those planning the way forward.

Appendix

Examples from the research reported by Brown and Harris (1978) of the severe events and ongoing difficulties that brought about depression in vulnerable women in Camberwell

Examples of difficulties: housing: overcrowded, damp, stressful (rows with landlord about noise) living conditions; rundown property in increasingly rough area; heavy traffic and parked lorries outside windows; inability to afford to maintain house, repairs, leaks, damp, etc. mounting; *work:* husband away three weeks per month at sea; strain and tension at work associated with takeover, plus long hours; *money:* divorced, and ill-health prevents work so constant struggle to manage budget; temporary unemployment of husband causing debts with threat of eviction; *children:* management difficulties with disturbed teenager; son addicted to drugs; backwardness and phenylketonuria in child requiring special diet and hospital visits; infertility; *marital:* infidelity of husband; husband drinks and gambles, rows with wife, etc.

Examples of events: constant rows with husband, left him after he assaulted her, was five months pregnant; mugged on way home – tried to strangle her; brother, who was seen by sister every two weeks, suddenly found out had cancer; heard that could not be rehoused for at least ten years unless moved out of city; boyfriend called off their engagement; found out husband was unfaithful; son announced he was emigrating; son diagnosed epileptic.

(Source: private communication)

Bibliography

Abramson, L. Y., Seligman, M. E. P. and Teasdale, J. D. (1978), 'Learned helplessness in humans: critique and reformulation', *Journal of Abnormal Psychology 87*, no. 1, pp. 49–74.

Adams, J. E. and Lindemann, E. (1974), 'Coping with long-term disability', in Coelho, G. V., Hamburg, D. A. and Adams, J. E. (eds), *Coping and Adaptation*, New York, Basic Books.

Ahrenfeldt, R. H. (1958), *Psychiatry in the British Army in the Second World War*, London, Routledge & Kegan Paul.

Akiskal, H. S. (1979), 'A biobehavioural approach to depression', in Depue, R. A. (ed.), *The Psychobiology of the Depressive Disorders: Implications for the Effects of Stress*, New York, Academic Press.

Antonovsky, A. (1979), *Health, Stress and Coping*, San Francisco, Jossey-Bass.

Arber, S., Gilbert, G. N. and Dale, A. (1985), 'Paid employment and women's health: a benefit or a source of role strain?', *Sociology of Health and Illness 7*, no. 3, pp. 375–400.

Aronowitz, E. (ed.) (1982), *Prevention Strategies for Mental Health*, published for Westchester County Dept of Community Mental Health, Prodist, New York.

Baldwin, J. A. (1977), 'Child abuse: epidemiology and prevention', in Graham, P. J. (ed.), *Epidemiological Approaches in Child Psychiatry*, London, Academic Press.

Banks, M. H. and Jackson, P. R. (1982), 'Unemployment and risk of minor psychiatric disorder in young people: cross-sectional and longitudinal evidence', *Psychological Medicine 12*, pp. 789–98.

Barnes, J. (ed.) (1975), 'Educational priority: curriculum innovation in London', *EPAs Vol. 3*, London, HMSO.

Barrowclough, C. and Tarrier, N. (1984), ' "Psychosocial" interventions with families and their effects on the course of schizophrenia: a review', *Psychological Medicine 14*, pp. 629–42.

Bateson, G., Jackson, D. D., Haley, J. and Weakland, J. H. (1956), 'Toward a theory of schizophrenia', *Behavioural Science 1*, pp. 251–64.

Bebbington, P., Hurry, J., Tennant, C., Sturt, E. and Wing, J. K. (1981), 'Epidemiology of mental disorders in Camberwell', *Psychological Medicine 11*, pp. 561–79.

Bebbington, P., Sturt, E., Tennant, C. and Hurry, J. (1984), 'Misfortune and resilience: a community study of women', *Psychological Medicine 14*, pp. 347–63.

Beck, A. T. (1973), *The Diagnosis and Management of Depression*, Philadelphia, University of Pennsylvania Press.

Beck, A., Ward, C. H., Mendelsohn, M., Mock, J. and Erbaugh, J. (1961), 'An inventory for measuring depression', *Archives of General Psychiatry 4*, pp. 561–71.

Beehr, T. A. (1976), 'Perceived situational moderators of the relationship between subjective role ambiguity and role strain', *Journal of Applied Psychology 61*, no. 1, pp. 35–40.

Beers, C. W. (1908), *A Mind that Found Itself*, New York, Longmans, Green.

Berkman, L. F. and Syme, S. L. (1979), 'Social networks, host resistance and mortality: a 9-year follow-up of Alameda County residents', *American Journal of Epidemiology 109*, no. 2, pp. 186–204.

Berkowitz, R., Eberlein-Fries, R., Kuipers, L. and Leff, J. (1984), 'Educating relatives about schizophrenia', *Schizophrenia Bulletin 10*, pp. 418–29.

Bifulco, A., Brown, G. W. and Harris, T. O. (1987), 'Childhood loss of parent, lack of adequate parental care and adult depression: a replication', *Journal of Affective Disorders*, *12*, pp. 115–18.

Birley, J. and Hudson, B. (1983), 'The family, the social network and rehabilitation', in Watts, F. N. and Bennett, D. H. (eds), *Theory and Practice of Psychiatric Rehabilitation*, Chichester, Wiley.

Birtchnell, J. (1970), 'Early parent death and mental illness', *British Journal of Psychiatry 116*, pp. 281–8.

Bloom, B. L. (1982), 'Advances and obstacles in prevention of mental disorders', in Schulberg, H. C. and Killilea, M. (eds), *The Modern Practice of Community Mental Health*, San Francisco, Jossey-Bass.

Bloom, B. L., Hodges, W. F. and Caldwell, R. A. (1982), 'A preventive program for the newly separated: initial evaluation', *American Journal of Community Psychology 10*, no. 3, pp. 251–64.

Bolton, W. and Oatley, K. (1987), 'A longitudinal study of social support and depression in unemployed men', *Psychological Medicine*, *17*, pp. 453–60.

Boulton, M. G. (1983), *On Being a Mother: A Study of Women with Pre-School Children*, London, Tavistock.

Bouras, N. and Tufnell, G. (1983), 'Mental Health Advice Centre: the crisis intervention team', Research Report no. 2, Lewisham and North Southwark Health Authority, London.

Bowlby, J. (1951), *Maternal Care and Mental Health*, Geneva, World Health Organisation.

Bowlby, J. (1969), *Attachment and Loss. Vol. 1: Attachment*, London, Hogarth Press.

Bowlby, J. (1973), *Attachment and Loss. Vol. 2: Separation, Anxiety and Anger*, London, Hogarth Press

Bowlby, J. (1980), *Attachment and Loss. Vol. 3: Loss, Sadness and Depression*, London, Hogarth Press.

Boyd, J. H. and Weissman, M. M. (1981), 'Epidemiology of affective disorders', *Archives of General Psychiatry 38*, pp. 1039–46.

Breakwell, G., Harrison, B. and Proper, C. (1982), 'The psychological benefits of YOPS', *New Society*, 23 September, pp. 494–5.

Brenner, M. H. (1973), *Mental Illness and the Economy*, Cambridge, Mass., Harvard University Press.

Bronfenbrenner, U. (1975), 'Is early intervention effective?', in Gultentag, M. and Struening, E. L. (eds), *Handbook of Evaluation Research*, Beverly Hills, Sage.

Brown, G. W. and Birley, J. L. T. (1968), 'Crisis and Life changes and the onset of schizophrenia', *Journal of Health and Social Behaviour 9*, pp. 203–14.

Brown, G. W. and Harris, T. O. (1978), *Social Origins of Depression*, London, Tavistock.

Brown, G. W. and Harris, T. (1986), 'Stressor, vulnerability and depression: a question of replication', editorial in *Psychological Medicine 16*, pp. 739–44.

Brown, G. W. and Rutter, M. (1966), 'The measurement of family activities and relationships: a methodological study', *Human Relations 19*, pp. 241–63.

Brown, G. W., Bone, M., Dalison, B. and Wing, J. K. (1966), *Schizophrenia and Social Care: A Comparative Follow-up of 339 Schizophrenic Patients*, Maudsley Monograph no. 17, London, Oxford University Press.

Brown, G. W., Birley, J. L. T. and Wing, J. K. (1972), 'Influence of family life on the course of schizophrenic disorders: a replication', *British Journal of Psychiatry 121*, pp. 241–58.

Brown, G. W., Craig, T. K. J. and Harris, T. O. (1985) 'Depression: distress or disease? Some epidemiological considerations', *British Journal of Psychiatry 147*, pp. 612–22.

Brown, G. W., Andrews, B., Harris, T., Adler, Z. and Bridge, L. (1986a), 'Social support, self-esteem and depression', *Psychological Medicine 16*, pp. 813–31.

Brown, G. W., Harris, T. O. and Bifulco, A. (1986b), 'Long-term effect of early loss of parent', in Rutter, M., Izard, C. and Read, P. (eds), *Depression in Childhood: Developmental Perspectives*, New York, Guildford Press.

Brown, G. W., Bifulco, A., Harris, T. and Bridge, L. (1986c), 'Life stress, chronic subclinical symptoms and vulnerability to clinical depression', *Journal of Affective Disorders 11*, pp. 1–19.

Brown, G. W., Bifulco, A. and Harris, T. O. (1987), 'Life events, vulnerability and onset of depression: some refinements', *British Journal of Psychiatry 150*, pp. 30–42.

Brown, P. (1985), *The Transfer of Care: Psychiatric Deinstitutionalization and its Aftermath*, London, Routledge & Kegan Paul.

Brownsberger, C. N., Seneriches, J. S., McDonagh, P. H., Yost, P. W., Bolton, C. F., Mutty, L. B. and Soloman, P. (1971), 'Common psychiatric symptoms', in Soloman, P. and Patch, V. *Handbook of Psychiatry*, 2nd edn, Los Altos, California, Lange.

Buckwald, A. M., Coyne, J. C. and Cole, C. S. (1978), 'A critical evaluation of the learned helplessness model of depression', *Journal of Abnormal Psychology 87*, no. 1, pp. 180–93.

Calloway, S. P., Dolan, R. J., Fonagy, P., De Souza, V. F. A. and Wakeling, A. (1984a), 'Endocrine changes and clinical profiles in depression: 1. The dexamethasone suppression test', *Psychological Medicine 14*, pp. 749–58.

Calloway S. P., Dolan, R. J., Fonagy, P., De Souza, V. F. A. and Wakeling, A. (1984b), 'Endocrine changes and clinical profiles in depression: 2. The thyrotopin-releasing hormone test', *Psychological Medicine 14*, pp. 759–65.

Cameron, J. and Parkes, C. M. (1983), 'Terminal care: evaluation of effects on surviving family of care before and after bereavement', *Postgraduate Medical Journal*, *59*, pp. 73–8.

Caplan, G. (1964), *Principles of Preventive Psychiatry*, New York, Basic Books.

Caplan-Moskovich, R. B. (1982), 'Gerald Caplan: the man and his work', in Schulberg, H. C. and Killilea, M. (eds), *The Modern Practice of Community Mental Health*, San Francisco, Jossey-Bass.

Cartwright, A. (1974), 'Exploratory studies of the services for maladjusted children', unpublished MPhil, University of London.

Cassel, J. (1976), 'The contribution of the social environment to host resistance', 4th Wade Hampton Frost lecture, *American Journal of Epidemiology 104*, no. 2, pp. 107–23.

Charter for Jobs (1985), 'We can cut unemployment', London, *Charter for Jobs, 1985* (PO Box 474, London, NW3).

Chazan, M. (1964), 'The incidence and nature of maladjustment among children in schools for the educationally subnormal', *British Journal of Educational Psychology 34*, pp. 292–304.

Child Development Project (1984), *Child Development Programme*, booklet produced by the University of Bristol.

Chu, F. D. and Trotter, S. (1974), *The Madness Establishment: Ralph Nader's Study Group Report on the National Institute of Mental Health*, New York, Grossman.

Clare, A. W. (1982), 'Social aspects of ill-health in general practice', in Clare, A. W. and Corney, R. H. (eds), *Social Work and Primary Health Care*, London, Academic Press.

Clare, A. W. and Corney, R. H. (eds) (1982), *Social Work and Primary Health Care*, London, Academic Press.

Cobb, S. (1976), 'Social support as a moderator of life stress', *Psychosomatic Medicine 38*, pp. 300–14.

Colarelli, N. O. and Siegel, S. M. (1966), *Ward H: An Adventure in Innovation*, New York, Van Nostrand.

Cooper, B. (1978), 'Epidemiology', in Wing, J. K. (ed.), *Schizophrenia: Toward a New Synthesis*, London, Academic Press.

Cooper, B. and Sosna, V. (1980), 'Family settings of the psychiatrically disturbed aged', in Robins, L. N., Clayton, P. J. and Wing J. K. (eds), *The Social Consequence of Psychiatric Illness*, New York, Brunner/Mazel.

Cooper, B., Harwin, B. G., Depla, C. and Shepherd, M. (1982), 'Mental health care in the community: an evaluative study', in Clare, A. W. and Corney, R. H. (eds), *Social Work and Primary Health Care*, London, Academic Press.

Cooper, C. L. (1980), 'Work and stress in white and blue-collar jobs', *Bulletin of the British Psychological Society 33*, pp. 49–51.

Cooper, J. E. (1979), *Crisis Admission Units and Emergency Psychiatric Services* (Public Health in Europe 11), Copenhagen, World Health Organisation, Regional Office for Europe.

Copeland, J. (1981), 'What is a case? A case for what?', in Wing, J. K., Bebbington, P. and Robins, L. N., *What is a Case?*, London, Grant McIntyre.

Corney, R. H. (1982), 'The effectiveness of social work intervention in the management of depressed women in general practice', in Clare, A. W. and Corney, R. H. (eds), *Social Work and Primary Health Care*, London, Academic Press.

Craig, T. K. J. and Brown, G. W. (1984), 'Life events, meaning and physical illness: a review', in Steptoe, A. and Mathews, A. (eds), *Health Care and Human Behaviour*, London, Academic Press.

Crook, S. and Wolkind, S. N. (1983), 'A longitudinal study of single mothers and their children', in Madge, N. (ed.), *Families at Risk*, London, Heinemann.

Crook, T. and Elliot, J. (1980), 'Parental death during childhood and adult depression: a critical review of the literature', *Psychology Bulletin 87*, pp. 252–9.

Cutting, J. (1985), *The Psychology of Schizophrenia*, Edinburgh, Churchill Livingstone.

Daniel, W. W. (1974), *A National Survey of the Unemployed*, London, Political and Economic Planning Institute Vol. 45, Broadsheet no. 546.

Dean, C., Surtees, P. G. and Sashidharan, S. P. (1983), 'Comparison of research diagnostic systems in an Edinburgh community sample', *British Journal of Psychiatry 142*, pp. 247–56.

Delozier, P. P. (1982), 'Attachment theory and child abuse', in Parkes, C. M. and Stevenson-Hinde, J. (eds), *The Place of Attachment in Human Behaviour*, New York, Basic Books.

DHSS (1974), *Report of the Committee of Inquiry into the Care and Supervision Provided in Relation to Maria Colwell* (Field-Fisher Report), London, HMSO.

DHSS (1977) *The Role of psychologists in the Health Service*, Report of a subcommittee on Mental Health chaired by Lord Trethowan, London, HMSO.

DHSS (1982), *Health and Personal Social Services Statistics for England 1982*, London, HMSO.

DHSS (1983) *In-Patient Statistics from the Mental Health Enquiry for England 1978*, Statistical and Research Report Series no. 24, London, HMSO.

Doane, J. A., West, K. L., Goldstein, M. J., Rodnick, E. H. and Jones, J. E. (1981), 'Parental communication deviance and affective style', *Archives of General Psychiatry 38*, pp. 679–85.

Dohrenwend, B. P. and Dohrenwend, B. S. (1969), *Social Status and Psychological Disorder: A Causal Enquiry*, New York, Wiley.

Dohrenwend, B. S. and Dohrenwend, B. P. (eds) (1974), *Stressful Life Events: Their Nature and Effects*, New York, Wiley.

Doll, R. (1983), 'Prospects for prevention', *British Medical Journal 286*, pp. 445–53.

Douglas, J. W. B. (1975), 'Early hospital admissions and later disturbances of behaviour and learning', *Develop. Med. Child Neurology 17*, pp. 456–80.

Durlak, J. A. and Jason, L. A. (1984), 'Preventive programs for school-aged children and adolescents', in Roberts, M. C. and Peterson, L. (eds), *Prevention of Problems in Childhood*, New York, Wiley.

Eales, M. J. (1985), 'Social factors in the occurrence of depression, and allied disorders, in unemployed men', unpublished PhD thesis, University of London.

Economic Intelligence Unit (1982), *Coping with Unemployment: the Effects on the Unemployed Themselves*, London, EIU.

Ellenberger, H. F. (1970), *The Discovery of the Unconscious: The History and Evolution of Dynamic Psychiatry*, New York, Basic Books.

Emery, A. E. H. (1975), *Elements of Medical Genetics*, 4th ed., Edinburgh, Churchill Livingstone.

Emery, A. E. H., Watt, M. S. and Clack, E. R. (1973), 'Social effects of genetic counselling', *British Medical Journal 1*, pp. 724–6.

Ennals, D. (1972), *Comment on the Robens Report and the Evidence Submitted by MIND*, London, MIND.

Epstein, S. (1983), 'Natural healing processes of the mind', in Meichenbaum, D. and Jaremko, M. E. (eds), *Stress Reduction and Prevention*, New York, Plenum Press.

Erlenmeyer-Kimling, L. (1979), 'Advantages of a behaviour-genetic approach to investigating stress in the depressive disorders', in Depue, R. A. (ed.), *The Psychobiology of the Depressive Disorders*, New York, Academic Press.

European Foundation for the Improvement of Living and Working Conditions (1981), *Physical and Psychological Stress at Work*, Document no. 2T 372, London, Tavistock Institute of Human Relations.

Eyken, W. van der (1982), *Homestart: A Four Year Evaluation*, Leicester, Homestart Consultancy.

Fagin, L. (1981), 'Unemployment and health in families (case studies based on family interviews – a pilot study), unpublished DHSS document.

Falloon, I. R. H., Boyd, J. L., McGill, C. W., Razani, J., Moss, H. and Gilderman, A. M. (1982), 'Family management in the prevention of exacerbations of schizophrenia', *New England Journal of Medicine 306*, pp. 1437–40.

Falloon, I. R. H., Boyd, J. L., McGill, C., Williamson, M., Razani, J., Moss, H. B., Gilderman, A. M. and Simpson, G. M. (1985), 'Family management in the prevention of morbidity of schizophrenia: clinical outcome of a two-year longitudinal study', *Archives of General Psychiatry 42*, pp. 887–96.

Felner, R. D., Ginter, M. and Primavera, J. (1982), 'Primary prevention during school transitions: social support and environmental structure', *American Journal of Community Psychology 10*, no. 3, pp. 277–90.

Ferguson, B. F. (1979), 'Preparing young children for hospitalisation: a comparison of two methods', *Pediatrics 64*, pp. 656–64.

Finlay-Jones, R. A. and Brown, G. W. (1981), 'Types of stressful life event and the onset of anxiety and depressive disorders', *Psychological Medicine 11*, pp. 803–15.

Fischer, M., Rolf, J. E., Hasazi, J. E. and Cummings, L. (1984), 'Follow-up of a preschool epidemiological sample: cross-age continuities and predictions of later adjustment with internalizing and externalizing dimensions of behaviour', *Child Development 55*, pp. 137–50.

Flaherty, E. W., Marecek, J., Olsen, K. and Wilcove, G. (1983), 'Preventing adolescent pregnancy: an interpersonal problem solving approach', *Prevention in Human Services 2*, no. 3, pp. 49–64.

Freeman, H. (1978), 'Pharmacological treatment and management', in J. K. Wing (ed.), *Schizophrenia: Towards a New Synthesis*, London, Academic Press.

Freeman, H. (1983), 'District psychiatric services: psychiatry for defined populations', in Bean, P. (ed.), *Mental Illness: Changes and Trends*, Chichester, Wiley.

Freeman, H. (1985), 'Training for community psychiatry', *Bulletin of the Royal College of Psychiatrists 9*, no. 2, pp. 29–32.

Freud, S. (1917), 'Mourning and melancholia', in Strachey, J. (ed.), *Completed Psychological Works*, vol. 14, London, Hogarth Press.

Garber, J., Miller, W. R. and Seamen, S. F. (1979), 'Learned helplessness, stress, and the depressive disorders', in Depue, R. A. (ed.), *The Psychobiology of Depressive Disorders*, New York, Academic Press.

Gavron, H. (1966), *The Captive Wife: Conflicts of Housebound Mothers*, London, Penguin.

Gelder, M. (1985), 'Cognitive therapy', in Granville-Grossman, K. (ed.) *Recent Advances in Clinical Psychiatry Vol. 5*, Edinburgh, Churchill Livingstone.

Gilbert, P. (1984), *Depression: From Psychology to Brain State*, London, Lawrence Erlbaum Associates.

Gillie, O., Price, A. and Robinson, S. (1982), *The Sunday Times Self-Help Directory*, 2nd edn., London, Granada.

Glasscote, R. M. (1980), *Preventing Mental Illness: Efforts and Attitudes*, Washington, DC, Joint Information Service.

Goldberg, D. (1972), *The Detection of Psychiatric Illness by Questionnaire*, Maudsley Monograph no. 21, London, Oxford University Press.

Goldberg, D. (1985), 'Identifying psychiatric illness among general medical patients', *British Medical Journal 291*, pp. 161-2.

Goldberg, D. and Blackwell, B. (1970), 'Psychiatric illness in general practice: a detailed study using a new method of case identification', *British Medical Journal 2*, pp. 439-43.

Goldberg, D. and Huxley, P. (1980), *Mental Illness in the Community: The Pathway to Psychiatric Care*, London, Tavistock;

Goldenberg, I. I. (1971), *Build Me a Mountain: Youth, Poverty, and the Creation of a New Setting*, Cambridge, Mass., MIT Press.

Goldstein, J., Freud, A. and Solnit, A. J. (1973), *Beyond the Best Interests of the Child*, New York, Free Press.

Goldstein, J., Freud, A. and Solnit, A. J. (1979), *Before the Best Interests of the Child*, New York, Free Press.

Goldthorpe, J. H. and Hope, K. (1974), *The Social Grading of Occupation: A New Approach and Scale*, Oxford, Clarendon Press.

Gore, S. (1978), 'The effect of social support in moderating the health consequences of unemployment', *Journal of Health and Social Behaviour 19*, pp. 157-65.

Gottesman, I. I. and Shields, J. (1972), *Schizophrenia and Genetics: A Twin Study Vantage Point*, New York, Academic Press.

Gottesman, I. I. and Shields, J. (1982), *Schizophrenia: The Epigenetic Puzzle*, Cambridge, Cambridge University Press.

Gottlieb, B. H. (1983), *Social Support Strategies: Guidelines for Mental Health Practice*, Beverly Hills, Sage.

Graham, M. (1983), Letter to Open Space, *Guardian*, 2 August.

Graham, P. J. (1977), 'Possibilities for prevention', in Graham, P. J. (ed.), *Epidemiological Approaches in Child Psychiatry*, London, Academic Press.

Graham, P. J. (1983), 'Problems of predicting disturbances in adulthood from behaviour disorders in childhood', in Russell, G. F. M. and Hersov, L. A. (eds), *Handbook of Psychiatry 4: The Neuroses and Personality Disorders*, Cambridge, Cambridge University Press.

Granville-Grossman, K. L. (1968), 'The early environment in affective disorder', in Coppen, A. and Walk, A. (eds), *Recent Developments in Affective Disorders*, *British Journal of Psychiatry* Special Publication no. 2.

Greer, S. (1985), 'Cancer: psychiatric aspects', in Granville-Grossman, K. (ed.), *Recent Advances in Clinical Psychiatry, Vol. 5*, Edinburgh, Churchill Livingstone.

Grosskurth, A. (1984), 'From care to nowhere', *Roof* (Shelter's housing magazine), July/August, pp. 11–14.

Gusella, J. F., Wexler, N. S., Conneally, P. M. *et al.* (1983), 'A polymorphic DNA marker genetically linked to Huntington's disease', *Nature 306*, pp. 234–8.

Harris, T. (1963), 'The social etiology of depression', in Korf, J. & Pepplinkhuizen L. (eds), *Depression: An Integrative View*, Proceedings of a symposium at Erasmus University, Rotterdam, The Netherlands, Drachten, TGO Foundation.

Harris, T., Brown, G. W. and Bifulco, A. (1986), 'Loss of parent in childhood and adult psychiatric disorder: the role of lack of adequate parental care', *Psychological Medicine 16*, pp. 641–59.

Harris, T., Brown, G. W. and Bifulco, A. (1987a), 'Loss of parent in childhood and adult psychiatric disorder: the role of social class position and premarital pregnancy', *Psychological Medicine 17*, no. 1, pp. 163–83.

Harris, T., Brown, G. W. and Bifulco, A. (1987b), 'Loss of parent in childhood and adult psychiatric disorder: the role of situational helplessness', MS.

Harris, T., Brown, G. W. and Bifulco, A. (1987c), 'A retrospective study of the link between childhood symptoms and depression in adulthood: the role of psycho-social factors', MS.

Henderson, S. (1974), 'Care eliciting behaviour in man', *Journal of Nervous and Mental Disease 159*, no. 3, pp. 172–81.

Henderson, S. (1982), 'The significance of social relationships in the aetiology of neurosis', in Parkes, C. M. and Stevenson Hinde, H. (eds), *The Place of Attachment in Human Behaviour*, London, Tavistock.

Henderson, S., Byrne, D. G., Duncan-Jones, P., Scott, R. and Adcock, S. (1980), 'Social relationships, adversity and neurosis: a study of associations in a general population sample', *British Journal of Psychiatry 136*, pp. 574–83.

Henderson, S., Byrne, D. G. and Duncan-Jones, P. (1981), *Neurosis and the Social Environment*, Sydney, Academic Press.

Hepworth, S. J. (1980), 'Moderating factors of the psychological impact of unemployment', *Journal of Occupational Psychology 53*, pp. 139–45.

Hetherington, E. M. (1979), 'Divorce: a child's perspective', *American Psychologist 34*, no. 10, pp. 851–8.

Hewison, J. and Tizard, J. (1980), 'Parental involvement and reading attainment', *British Journal of Educational Psychology 50*, pp. 209–15.

Hirsch, S. R. and Leff, J. P. (1975), *Abnormalities in Parents of Schizophrenics*, Institute of Psychiatry, Maudsley Monograph no. 22, London, OUP.

Hoeper, E. W., Kessler, L. G., Nycz, G. R., Burke, J. D. and Pierce, W. E. (1984), 'The usefulness of screening for mental illness', *Lancet 1*, pp. 33–5.

Holmes, T. H. and Rahe, R. (1967), 'The social readjustment rating scale', *Journal of Psychosomatic Research 11*, pp. 213–18.

House, J. S. (1981), *Work Stress and Social Support*, Reading, Mass., Addison-Wesley.

House, R. J. and Rizzo, J. R. (1972), 'Role conflict and ambiguity as critical variables in a model of organisational behaviour', *Organisational Behaviour and Human Performance 7*, pp. 467–505.

Jahoda, M. (1979), 'The psychological meanings of unemployment', *New Society*, 6 September, pp. 492–5.

Jaremko, M. E. (1983), 'Stress inoculation training for social anxiety, with emphasis on dating anxiety', in Meichenbaum, D. and Jaremko, M. E. (eds), *Stress Reduction and Prevention*, New York, Plenum Press.

Jerrom, D. W. A., Simpson, R. J., Barber, J. H. and Pemberton, D. A. (1983), 'General Practitioners' satisfaction with a primary care clinical psychology service' *Journal of the Royal College of General Practitioners 33*, pp. 29–31.

Johnson, D. L. and Breckenridge, J. N. (1982), 'The Houston Parent and Child Development Center and the primary prevention of behaviour problems in young children', *American Journal of Community Psychology 10*, no. 3, pp. 305–16.

Johnson, J. E. (1984), 'Psychological interventions and coping with surgery', in Baum, A., Taylor, S. E. and Singer, J. E. (eds), *Handbook of Psychology and Health, Vol. IV*, New Jersey, Lawrence Erlbaum Associates.

Johnson, J. H. and Sarason, I. G. (1978), 'Life stress, depression and anxiety: internal-external control as a moderator variable', *Journal of Psychosomatic Research 22*, pp. 205–8.

Johnstone, A. and Goldberg, D. (1976), 'Psychiatric screening in general practice', *Lancet 1*, pp. 606–8.

Jones, L., Simpson, D., Brown, A. C., Bainton, D. and McDonald, H. (1984), 'Prescribing psychotropic drugs in general practice: 3-year study', *British Medical Journal 289*, pp. 1045–8.

Kahn, R. L. and French, J. R. P. (1962), 'The effects of occupational status and health', *Journal of Social Issues 18*, no. 3, pp. 67–89.

Kahn, R. L. and French, J. R. P. (1970), 'Status and conflict: two themes in the study of stress', in McGrath, J. E. (ed.), *Social and Psychological Factors in Stress*, New York, Holt, Rinehart & Winston.

Karasek, R. A. (1979), 'Job demands, job description latitude, and mental strain: implications for job redesign', *Admin. Sc. Quarterly 24*, no. 2, pp. 285–308.

Kasl, S. V. (1984), 'Chronic life stress and health', in Steptoe, A. and Mathews, A. (eds), *Health Care and Human Behaviour*, London, Academic Press.

Kennedy, S., Thompson, R., Stancer, H. C., Roy, A. and Perzad, E. (1983), 'Life events precipitating mania', *British Journal of Psychiatry 142*, pp. 398–403.

Kessler, R. C. and McLeod, J. (1984), 'Social support and psychological distress in community surveys', in Cohen, S. and Syme, L. (eds), *Social Support and Health*, New York, Academic Press.

Kessler, R. C. and McRae, J. A. (1981), 'Trends in the relationship between sex and psychological distress: 1957–76', *American Sociological Review 46*, pp. 443–52.

Kestenbaum, C. J. (1980), 'Children at risk from schizophrenia', *American Journal of Psychotherapy 34*, no. 2, pp. 164–77.

Kolvin, I., Garside, R. F., Nicol, A. R., Macmillan, A., Wolstenholme, F. and Leitch, I. M. (1981), *Help Starts Here*, London, Tavistock.

Kreitman, N. (1983), 'Suicide and parasuicide', in Kendell, R. E. and Zealley, A. K. (eds), *Companion to Psychiatric Studies*, Edinburgh, Churchill Livingstone.

Lamb, H. R. and Zusman, J. (1979), 'Primary prevention in perspective', *American Journal of Psychiatry 136*, no. 1, pp. 12–17.

Lancet (1984), 'Towards better general practice', editorial, *Lancet 2*, pp. 1436–8.

Langner, T. S. and Michael, S. T. (1963), *Life Stress and Mental Health*, London, Free Press.

Lazar, I., Darlington, R., Murray, H., Royce, J. and Snipper, A. (1982), 'Lasting effects of early education: a report from the consortium for Longitudinal Studies', *Monographs of the Society for Research in Child Development*, serial no. 195, *47*, pp. 2–3.

Lazarus, R. S. (1976), *Patterns of Adjustment*, New York, McGraw-Hill.

Lazarus, R. S. and Cohen, J. B. (1977), 'Environmental stress', in Altman I. and Wohlwill, J. (eds), *Human Behaviour and the Environment Vol. 1*, New York, Plenum Press.

Leach, P. (1979), *Who Cares?* Harmondsworth, Penguin.

Leff, J. (1985), 'Family treatment of schizophrenia', in Granville-Grossman, K. (ed.), *Recent Advances in Clinical Psychiatry No. 5*, Edinburgh, Churchill Livingstone.

Leff, J. P. and Vaughn, C. E. (1980), 'The influence of life events and relatives' expressed emotion in schizophrenia and depressive neurosis', *British Journal of Psychiatry 136*, pp. 146–53.

Leff, J. P. and Vaughn, C. E. (1981), 'The role of maintenance therapy and relatives' expressed emotion in relapse of schizophrenia: a two-year follow-up', *British Journal of Psychiatry 139*, pp. 102–4.

Leff, J. P. and Vaughn, C. E. (1985), *Expressed Emotion in Families: Its Significance for Mental Illness*, London, Guildford.

Leff, J., Kuipers, L., Berkowitz, R., Eberlein-Vries, R. and Sturgeon, D. (1982), 'A controlled trial of social intervention in the families of schizophrenia patients', *British Journal of Psychiatry 141*, pp. 121–34.

Leff, J., Kuipers, L., Berkowitz, R. and Sturgeon, D. (1985), 'A controlled trial of social intervention in the families of schizophrenia patients: two-year follow-up', *British Journal of Psychiatry 146*, pp. 594–600.

Leff, J. P., Wig, N., Ghosh, A., Bedi, H., Menon, D. K., Kuipers, L., Korten, A., Ernberg, G., Day, R., Sartorius, N. and Jablensky, A. (1987), 'The influence of relatives' expressed emotion on the course of schizophrenia in Chandigarh', *British Journal of Psychiatry* (in press).

Leighton, A. (1982), *Caring for Mentally Ill People: Psychological and Social Barriers in a Historical Context*, Cambridge, Cambridge University Press.

Levi, L. (1979), 'Occupational mental health: its monitoring, protection and promotion', *Journal of Occupational Medicine 21*, no. 1, pp. 26–32.

Levi, L. (1981), *Preventing Work Stress*, Reading, Mass., Addison Wesley.

Levine, M. (1981), *The History and Politics of Community Mental Health*, New York, Oxford University Press.

Lewis, M., Feiring, C., McGuftog, C. and Jaskir, J. (1984), 'Predicting psychopathology in 6-year-olds from early social relations', *Child Development 55*, pp. 123–36.

Lin, N., Ensel, W. M., Simeone, R. S. and Kuo, W. (1979), 'Social support, stressful life events and illness: a model and an empirical test', *Journal of Health and Social Behaviour 20*, pp. 108–19.

Lloyd, G. G. (1985), 'Emotional aspects of physical illness', in Granville-Grossman, K. (ed.), *Recent Advances in Clinical Psychiatry Vol. 5*, Edinburgh, Churchill Livingstone.

Lofquist, L. M. and Davis, R. V. (1969), *Adjustment and Work*, New York, Appleton.

McGuire, M. and Sifneos, P. E. (1970), 'Problem-solving in psychotherapy', *Psychiatric Quarterly 44*, pp. 667–73.

Maguire, P. Tait, A., Brooke, M. Thomas, C. and Sellwood, R. (1980), 'The effect of counselling on the psychiatric morbidity associated with mastectomy', *British Medical Journal 281*, pp. 1454–6.

Maguire, P., Brooke, M., Tait, A., Thomas, C. and Sellwood, R. (1983), 'The effect of counselling on physical disability and social recovery after mastectomy', *Clinical Oncology 9*, pp. 319–24.

Marsh, G. and Meacher, M. (1979), 'The primary health care team: the way forward for mental health care', in Meacher, M. (ed.), *New Methods of Mental Health Care*, Oxford, Pergamon Press.

Mechanic, D. (1970), 'Some problems in developing a social psychology of adaptation to stress', in McGrath, J. E. (ed.), *Social and Psychological Factors in Stress*, New York, Holt, Rinehart & Winston.

Mechanic, D. (1986), 'The role of social factors in health and well-being: the biopsychosocial model from a social perspective', *Integrative Psychiatry* (in press).

Mednick, A., Schulsinger, F. and Venables, P. H. (1981a), 'A fifteen-year follow-up of children with schizophrenic mothers' (Denmark), in Mednick, S. A. and Baert, A. E. (eds), *Prospective Longitudinal Research: An Empirical Basis for the Primary Prevention of Psychosocial Disorders*, Oxford, Oxford University Press on behalf of WHO Regional Office for Europe.

Mednick, S. A., Schulsinger, F. and Venables, P. H. (1981b), 'The Mauritius Project', in Mednick, S. A. and Baert, A. E., (eds), *Prospective Longitudinal Research: An Empirical Basis for the Primary Prevention of Psychosocial Disorders*, Oxford, Oxford University Press on behalf of WHO Regional Office for Europe.

Meichenbaum, D. H. (1972), 'Cognitive modification of test-anxious college students', *Journal of Consulting and Clinical Psychology 39*, pp. 370–80.

Meichenbaum, D. H. (1977), *Cognitive-Behaviour Modification: An Integrative Approach*, New York, Plenum Press.

Meichenbaum, D. and Jaremko, M. E. (eds) (1983), *Stress Reduction and Prevention*, New York, Plenum Press.

Meyer, R. J. and Haggerty, R. J. (1962), 'Streptococcal infection in families: factors altering individual susceptibility', *Pediatrics 29*, pp. 539–49.

Miles, I. (1983), 'Is unemployment a health hazard?', *New Scientist*, 12 May, pp. 384–6.

Mills, M., Puckering, C., Pound, A. and Cox, A. D. (1985), 'What is it about depressed mothers that influences their children's functioning?', in Stevenson, J. E. (ed.), 'Book Supplement' to *Journal of Child Psychology and Psychiatry*, no. 4.

MIND (1971), *Stress at Work*, London, Mind Report no. 3.

Minturn, L. and Lambert, W. L. (1964), *Mothers of Six Cultures: Antecedents of Child Rearing*, New York, Wiley.

Mitchell, A. R. K. (1985), 'Psychiatrists in primary health care settings', *British Journal of Psychiatry 147*, pp. 371–9.

Moylem, S. and Davies, R. (1980), 'The disadvantages of the unemployed', *Employment Gazettes 88*, no. 8, pp. 830–2.

Murphy, E. (1983), 'The prognosis of depression in old age', *British Journal of Psychiatry 142*, pp. 111–19.

Murphy, H. B. M. (1983), 'Sociocultural variations in symptomatology, incidence and course of illness', in Shepherd, M. and Sangwill, O. L. (eds), *Handbook of Psychiatry Vol. I: General Psychopathology*, Cambridge, Cambridge University Press.

National Council for Mental Hygiene (1927), 'The probable causes of mental disorder', Appendix to the *Fourth Report of the National Council for Mental Hygiene* (1926/7).

National Mental Health Association (1986), *The Prevention of Mental-Emotional Disabilities*, Alexandria, Virginia, NMHA.

Neighbors, H. W., Jackson, J. S., Bowman, P. J. and Gurin, G. (1983), 'Stress, coping and black mental health: preliminary findings from a national study', *Prevention in Human Services 2*, no. 3, pp. 5–29.

Nelson, G. (1982), 'Parental death during childhood and adult depression: some additional data', *Social Psychiatry 17*, pp. 37–42.

Newman, J. E. and Beehr, T. A. (1979), 'Personal and organisational strategies for handling job stress: a review of research and opinion', *Personnel Psychology 32*, pp. 1–42.

Newton, J. and Robinson, J. (1982), *Special School Leavers: The Value of Further Education in their Transition to the Adult World*, London, Greater London Association for the Disabled.

Oakley, A. (1974), *The Sociology of Housework*, Oxford, Martin Robertson.

O'Connor, P. and Brown, G. W. (1984), 'Supportive relationships: fact or fancy?', *Journal of Social and Personal Relationships 1*, pp. 159–75.

Osofsky, H. J., Osofsky, J. D., Kendall, V. and Rajan, R. (1973), 'Adolescents as mothers: an interdisciplinary approach to a complete problem', *Journal of Youth and Adolescence 2*, pp. 233–49.

Parkes, C. M. (1972), *Bereavement: Studies of Grief in Adult Life*, London, Tavistock.

Parkes, C. M. (1975), 'Determinants of outcome following bereavement', *Omega 6*, pp. 303–23.

Parkes, C. M. (1980), 'Bereavement counselling: does it work?', *British Medical Journal 281*, pp. 3–6.

Parkes, C. M. (1981), 'Evaluation of a bereavement service', *Journal of Preventive Psychiatry 1*, no. 2, pp. 179–88.

Parkes, C. M. (1982a), 'Role of support systems in loss and psychosocial transitions', in Schulberg, H. C. and Killilea, M. (eds), *The Modern Practice of Community Mental Health*, San Francisco, Jossey-Bass.

Parkes, C. M. (1982b), 'Attachment and the prevention of mental disorders', in Parkes, C. M. and Stevenson-Hinde, J. (eds), *The Place of Attachment in Human Behaviour*, London, Tavistock.

Parkes, C. M. and Brown, R. J. (1972), 'Health after bereavement: a controlled study of young Boston widows and widowers', *Psychosomatic Medicine 34*, no. 5, pp. 449–61.

Parkes, C. M. and Weiss, R. S. (1983), *Recovery from Bereavement*, New York, Basic Books.

Parkinson, L. (1982), 'Bristol Family Courts', *Association of Child Psychology and Psychiatry Newsletter*, report no. 11.

Parnas, J., Schulsinger, F., Schulsinger, H., Mednick, S. A. and Teasdale, T. T. (1982), 'Behavioral precursors of schizophrenia spectrum', *Archives of General Psychiatry 39*, pp. 658–64.

Parry, G. (1986), 'Paid employment, life events, social support and mental health in working-class mothers', *Journal of Health and Social Behaviour 27*, pp. 193–208.

Paykel, E. S. (1978), 'Contribution of life events to causation of psychiatric illness', *Psychological Medicine 8*, pp. 245–53.

Paykel, E. S. (1979), 'Recent life events in the development of the depressive disorders', in Depue, R. A. (ed.), *The Psychobiology of the Depressive Disorders*, London, Academic Press.

Paykel, E. S., Rao, B. M. and Taylor, C. N. (1984), 'Life stress and symptom pattern in out-patient depression', *Psychological Medicine 14*, pp. 559–68.

Pearlin, L. I. and Schooler, C. (1978), 'The structure of coping', *Journal of Health and Social Behaviour 19*, pp. 2–21.

Pearlin, L. I., Menaghan, E. G., Lieberman, M. A. and Mullen, J. R. (1981), 'The stress process', *Journal of Health and Social Behaviour 22*, pp. 337–56.

Peterson, L. and Brownlee-Duffeck, M. (1984), 'Prevention of anxiety and pain due to medical and dental procedures', in Roberts, M. C. and Peterson, L. (eds), *Prevention of Problems in Childhood*, New York, Wiley.

Platt, S. D. (1984), 'Unemployment and suicidal behaviour: a review of the literature', *Social Science and Medicine, 19*, pp. 93–115.

Platt, S. D. and Kreitman, N. (1984), 'Trends in parasuicide and unemployment among men in Edinburgh, 1968–82', *British Medical Journal 289*, pp. 1029–32.

Potter Lee N. and West, K. (1979), 'Assertion training', paper to MIND's Annual Conference *Prevention in Mental Health*, London, MIND.

Pound, A. and Mills, M. (1983), 'The impact of maternal depression on young children', paper presented at the Tavistock Centre Scientific Meeting, London, 10 January.

Pound, A., Mills, M. and Cox, T. (1985), 'A pilot evaluation of Newpin. A home-visiting and befriending scheme in south London', MS, summarised in the October *Newsletter of the Association of Child Psychology and Psychiatry*.

Price, J. (1968), 'The genetics of depressive behaviour', in Coppen, A. and Walk, A. (eds), *Recent Developments in Affective Disorders, British Journal of Psychiatry Special Publication no. 2*.

Pritchard, P. (1981), *Manual of Primary Health Care*, Oxford, Oxford University Press.

Quinton, D. and Rutter, M. (1976), 'Early hospital admissions and later disturbances of behaviour: an attempted replication of Douglas' findings', *Develop. Med. Child Neurology 18*, pp. 447–58.

Quinton, D. and Rutter, M. (1983), 'Parenting behaviour of mothers raised "in care" ', in Nicol, A. R. (ed.), *Practical Lessons from Longitudinal Studies*, Chichester, Wiley.

Quinton, D. and Rutter, M. (1984a), 'Parents with children in care. I. Current circumstances and parenting', *Journal of Child Psychology and Psychiatry 25*, pp. 211–29.

Quinton, D. and Rutter, M. (1984b), 'Parents with children in care. II. Intergenerational continuities', *Journal of Child Psychology and Pychiatry 25*, pp. 231–50.

Quinton, D., Rutter, M. and Liddle, C. (1984), 'Institutional rearing, parenting difficulties and marital support', *Psychological Medicine 14*, pp. 107–24.

Raphael, B. (1977), 'Preventive intervention with the recently bereaved', *Archives of General Psychiatry 34*, p. 1450–4.

Raphael, B. (1982), 'The young child and the death of a parent', in Parkes, C. M. and Stevenson-Hinde, J. (eds), *The Place of Attachment in Human Behaviour*, London, Tavistock.

Ratna, L. (1978), *The Practice of Psychiatric Crisis Intervention*, 2nd Edn, St Albans, League of Friends, Napsbury Hospital.

Rawnsley, K. (1968), 'Epidemiology of affective disorder', in Coppen, A. and Walk, A. (eds), *Recent Developments in Affective Disorders*, British Journal of Psychiatry Special Publication no. 2.

Richardson, A. and Goodman, M. (1983), *Self-Help and Social Care: Mutual Aid Organisations in Practice*, London, Policy Studies Institute/DHSS.

Richman, A. and Barry, A. (1985), 'More and more is less and less: the myth of massive psychiatric need', *British Journal of Psychiatry 146*, pp. 164–8.

Richman, N. (1978), 'Depression in mothers of young children', *Journal of Royal Society of Medicine 71*, pp. 489–93.

Richman, N., Stevenson, J. and Graham, P. J. (1982), *Preschool to School: A Behavioral Study*, London, Academic Press.

Rickel, A. U., Dyhdalo, L. L. and Smith, R. L. (1984), 'Prevention with preschoolers', in Roberts, M. C. and Peterson, L. (eds), *Prevention of Problems in Childhood*, New York, Wiley.

Robens, A. (Chairman) (1972), *Report of the Committee on Health and Safety at Work*, London, HMSO.

Roberts, M. C. and Peterson, L. (1984), 'Prevention models: theoretical and practical implications', in Roberts, M. C. and Peterson, L. (eds), *Prevention of Problems in Childhood*, New York, Wiley.

Robins, E. (1981), *The Final Months: A Study of the Lives of 134 Persons who Committed Suicide*, Oxford, Oxford University Press.

Robins, L. N. (1966), *Deviant Children Grown Up*, Baltimore, William & Wilkins.

Robins, L. N. (1978), 'Psychiatric epidemiology', *Archives of General Psychiatry 35*, p. 697.

Robins, L. N. and Ratcliff, K. S. (1980), 'Childhood conduct disorders and later arrest', in Robins, L. N., Clayton, P. J. and Wing, J. K. (eds), *The Social Consequences of Psychiatric Illness*, New York, Brunner/Mazel.

Rodin, J. (1983), 'Behavioural medicine: beneficial effects of self-control training in aging', *International Review of Applied Psychology 32*, pp. 153–81.

Rodin, J. (1985), 'Health, control and aging', in Baltes, M. M. and Baltes, P. B. (eds), *Aging and the Psychology of Control*, Hillsdale, New Jersey, Lea.

Rosenthal, D. (1968), 'Summary of the conference', in Rosenthal, D. and Kety, S. S. (eds), *Transmission of Schizophrenia*, Oxford, Pergamon Press.

Royal College of General Practitioners (1972), *The Future General Practitioner: Learning and Teaching*, Report of a working party, London, RCGP.

Royal College of General Practitioners (1981a), 'Health and prevention in primary care', *Report from General Practice 18*, London, RCGP.

Royal College of General Practitioners, (1981b), 'Prevention of arterial disease in general practice', *Report from General Practice 19*, London, RCGP.

Royal College of General Practitioners, (1981c), 'Prevention of psychiatric disorders in general practice', *Report from General Practice 20*, London, RCGP.

Royal College of General Practitioners (1981d), 'Family planning: an exercise in preventive medicine', *Report from General Practice 21*, London, RCGP.

Royal College of General Practitioners (1982), 'Healthier children: thinking prevention', *Report from General Practice 22*, London, RCGP.

Royal College of Psychiatrists (1983), Evidence prepared for the Social Services Committee on *Children in Care* (Chairman Renee Short), London, HMSO.

Rutter, M. L. (1966), *Children of Sick Parents: An Environmental and Psychiatric Study*, Maudsley Monograph no. 16, London, Oxford University Press.

Rutter, M. L. (1977), 'Brain damage syndromes in childhood: concepts and findings', *Journal of Child Psychology and Psychiatry 18*, pp. 1–21.

Rutter, M. L. (1979a), 'Protective factors in children's responses to stress and disadvantage', in Kent, M. W. and Rolf, J. E. (eds), *Primary Prevention of Psychopathology, Vol. 3: Social Competence in Children*, Hanover, New Hampshire, University Press of New England.

Rutter, M. L. (1979b), 'Separation experiences: a new look at an old topic', *Journal of Pediatrics 95*, no. 1, pp. 147–154.

Rutter, M. L. (1981), *Maternal Deprivation Reassessed*, Harmondsworth, Penguin.

Rutter, M. L. (1982), 'Prevention of children's psychosocial disorders: myth and substance', *Pediatrics 70*, no. 6, pp. 883–94.

Rutter, M. L. (1985), 'Resilience in the face of adversity: protective factors and resistance to psychiatric disorder', *British Journal of Psychiatry 147*, pp. 598–611.

Rutter, M. L. and Madge, N. (1976), *Cycles of Disadvantage*, London, Heinemann.

Rutter, M. L., Tizard, J. and Whitmore, J. (1970), *Education, Health and Behaviour*, London, Longman.

Rutter, M. L., Cox, A., Tupling, C., Berger, M. and Yule, W. (1975a), 'Attainment and adjustment in two geographical areas: I. The prevalence of psychiatric disorder', *British Journal of Psychiatry 126*, pp. 493–509.

Rutter, M. L., Yule, B., Quinton, D., Rowlands, O., Yule, W. and Berger, M. (1975b), 'Attainment and adjustment in two geographical areas: III. Some factors accounting for area differences', *British Journal of Psychiatry 126*, pp. 520–33.

Rutter, M. L., Maughan, B., Mortimer, P. and Ousten, J. (1979), *Fifteen Thousand Hours: Secondary Schools and their Effects on Children*, London, Open Books.

Rutter, M. L., Quinton, D. and Liddle, C. (1983), 'Parenting in two generations: looking backwards and looking forwards', in Madge, N. (ed.), *Families at Risk*, London, SSRC/DHSS/Heinemann.

Sainsbury, P. (1968), 'Suicide and depression', in Coppen, A. and Walk, A. (eds), *Recent Developments in Affective Disorders*, *British Journal of Psychiatry*, Special Publication no. 2.

Sainsbury, P. (1973), 'A comparative evaluation of a comprehensive community psychiatric service', in Cawley, R. and McLachlan, G. (eds), *Policy for Action*, Oxford, Oxford University Press.

Salmon, A. (1985), 'The haunted heroes', film for BBC television, screened BBC2, 13 October.

Sampson, O. C. (1980), *Child Guidance: Its History, Provenance and Future*, London, British Psychological Society.

Sarason, S. B. (1972), *The Creation of Settings and the Future Societies*, San Francisco, Jossey-Bass.

Schaeffer, M., Kliman, G., Friedman, H. and Pasquariella, B. (1982), 'Children in foster care: a preventive service and research program for a high risk population', in Aronowitz, E. (ed.), *Prevention Strategies for Mental Health*, New York, Prodist.

Schulz, R. (1976), 'Effects of control and predictability on the physical and psychological well-being of the institutionalised aged', *Journal of Personality and Social Psychology 33*, no. 5, pp. 563–73.

Seebohm, F. (Chairman) (1968), *Report of the Committee on Local Authority and Allied Personal Social Services*, Cmnd 3703, London, HMSO.

Seligman, M. E. P. (1975), *Helplessness: On Depression, Development and Death*, San Francisco, Freeman.

Shaffer, D. (1983), 'Classification of psychiatric disorders in children', in Russell, G. F. M. and Hersov, L. A. (eds), *Handbook of Psychiatry 4: The Neuroses and Personality Disorders*, Cambridge, Cambridge University Press.

Shepherd, M., Cooper, B., Brown, A. C. and Kalton, G. W. (1966), *Psychiatric Illness in General Practice*, London, Oxford University Press.

Sheppard, M. G. (1983), 'Referrals from general practitioners to a social services department', *Journal of Royal College of General Practitioners 33*, pp. 33–9.

Shimmin, S., McNally, J. and Liff, S. (1981), 'Pressures on women engaged in factory work', *Employment Gazette*, August, pp. 344–9.

Shure, M. B. and Spivack, G. (1982), 'Interpersonal problem solving in young children: a cognitive approach to prevention', *American Journal of Community Psychology 10*, no. 3, pp. 341–56.

Silver, R. and Wortman, C. (1980), 'Coping with undesirable life events', in Garber, J. and Seligman, M. E. P. (eds), *Human Helplessness*, New York, Academic Press.

Singer, M. T. and Wynne, L. C. (1966), 'Communication styles in parents of normals, neurotics and schizophrenics', *Psychiat. Res. Rep. 20*, pp. 25–38.

Smith, R. (1985), ' "I'm just not right": the physical health of the unemployed', *British Medical Journal 291*, pp. 1626–9.

Smith, R. (1986a), 'Occupationless health: what can be done?: responding to unemployment and health', *British Medical Journal 292*, pp. 263–5.

Smith, R. (1986b), 'Occupationless health: training and "work" for the unemployed', *British Medical Journal 292*, pp. 320–3.

Smith, R. (1986c), 'Occupationless health: improving the health of the unemployed: a job for the health authorities and health workers', *British Medical Journal 292*, pp. 470–2.

Spitzer, R. L., Endicott, J. and Robins, E. (1978), 'Research diagnostic criteria: rationale and reliability', *Archives of General Psychiatry 35*, pp. 773–82.

Stafford, E. M. (1982), 'The impact of the Youth Opportunities Programme on young people's employment prospects and psychological well-being', *British Journal Guidance and Counselling 10*, no. 1, pp. 12–21.

Strathdee, G. and Williams, P. (1984), 'A survey of psychiatrists in primary care: the silent growth of a new service', *Journal of the Royal College of General Practitioners 34*, pp. 615–18.

Strauss, J. S. and Carpenter, W. T. (1981), *Schizophrenia*, New York, Plenum Press.

Strole, L., Langner, T. S., Michael, S. T., Opler, M. K. and Rennie, T. A. C. (1962), *Mental Health in the Metropolis*, New York, McGraw-Hill.

Surtees, P. G., Dean, C., Ingham, J. G., Kreitman, N. B., Miller, P. McC. and Sashidharan, S. P. (1983), 'Psychiatric disorder in women from an Edinburgh community: associations with demographic factors', *British Journal of Psychiatry 142*, pp. 238–46.

Sylva, K. (1983), 'Some lasting effects on pre-school – or the Emperor wore clothes after all', *British Psychological Society Education Section Review 1*, pp. 10–16.

Tableman, B., Marciniak, D., Johnson, D. and Rodgers, R. (1982), 'Stress management training for women on public assistance', *American Journal of Community Psychology 10*, no. 3, pp. 357–67.

Tennant, C. and Andrews, G. (1978), 'The pathogenic quality of life event stress in neurotic impairment', *Archives of General Psychiatry 35*, pp. 859–63.

Tennant, C., Bebbington, P. and Hurry, J. (1981), 'The role of life events in depressive illness: is there a substantial causal relation?', *Psychological Medicine 11*, pp. 379–89.

Test, M. and Stein, L. (1978), 'Training in community living: research design and results', in Stein, L. and Test, M. (eds), *Alternatives to Mental Hospital Treatment*, New York, Plenum Press.

Thomas, A. and Chess, S. (1977), *Temperament and Development*, New York, Brunner/Mazel.

Toynbee, P. (1983), 'The counsellor in the doctor's chair', *Guardian*, 25 July.

Vaughn, C. E. and Leff, J. P. (1976), 'The influence of family and social factors on the course of psychiatric illness: a comparison of schizophrenic and depressed neurotic patients', *British Journal of Psychiatry 129*, pp. 125–37.

Venables, P. H. (1964), 'Performance and level of activation in schizophrenics and normals', *British Journal of Psychiatry 55*, pp. 207–18.

Wallace, M. (1985), 'When freedom is a life sentence', *The Times*, 16 December.

Wallerstein, J. S. (1984), 'Children of divorce: preliminary report of a 10-year follow-up of young children' *American Journal of Orthopsychiatry 54*, no. 3, pp. 444–58.

Warner, R. (1985), *Recovery from Schizophrenia: Psychiatry and Political Economy*, London, Routledge & Kegan Paul.

Warr, P. (1984), 'Job loss, unemployment and psychological well-being', in Allen, V. L. and Vliert, E. van de (eds), *Role Transitions*, New York, Plenum Press.

Weiss, R. S. (1982), 'Relationship of social support and psychological well-being', in Schulberg, H. C. and Killilea, M. (eds), *The Modern Practice of Community Mental Health*, San Francisco, Jossey-Bass.

Weissman, M. M. and Klerman, G. L. (1978), 'Epidemiology of mental disorders', *Archives of General Psychiatry 35*, pp. 705–15.

Wells, N. (1983), *Teenage Mothers*, Liverpool, Children's Research Fund.

Williams, P. and Clare, A. (1981), 'Changing patterns of psychiatric care', *British Medical Journal 282*, pp. 375–7.

Wing, J. K. (1980), 'Methodological issues in psychiatric case identification', *Psychological Medicine 10*, pp. 5–10.

Wing, J. K. and Brown, G. W. (1970), *Institutionalisim and Schizophrenia*, Cambridge, Cambridge University Press.

Wing, J. K., Bennett, D. H. and Denham, J. (1964), 'Industrial rehabilitation of

long-stay schizophrenic patients', Medical Research Council memorandum no.
42, London, HMSO.

Wing, J. K., Cooper, J. E. and Sartorius, N. (1974), *The Measurement and Classification of Psychiatric Symptoms*, Cambridge, Cambridge University Press.

Wing, J. K., Mann, S. A., Leff, J. T. and Nixon, J. N. (1978), 'The concept of a case in psychiatric population surveys', *Psychological Medicine 8*, pp. 203–19.

Wing, J. K. and Sturt, E. (1978), *The PSE-ID-CATEGO System Supplementary Manual*, London, Medical Research Council Social Psychiatry Unit.

Wolfer, J. A. and Visintainer, M. A. (1979), 'Prehospital psychological preparation for tonsillectomy patients: effects on children's and parents' adjustment, *Pediatrics 64*, pp. 646–55.

Wolff, S. (1983a), 'Determinants of emotional and conduct disorders in childhood', in Russell, G. F. M. and Hersov, L. A. (eds), *Handbook of Psychiatry 4: The Neuroses and Personality Disorders*, Cambridge, Cambridge University Press.

Wolff, S. (1983b), 'The impact of sociopathic and inadequate parents on their children (including child abuse)', in Russell, G. F. M. and Hersov, L. A. (eds), *Handbook of Psychiatry 4: The Neuroses and Personality Disorders*, Cambridge, Cambridge University Press.

Wolkind, S. N. (1974), 'The components of "affectionless psychopathy" in institutionalised children', *Journal of Child Psychology and Psychiatry 15*, pp. 215–20.

Wolkind, S. N., Hall, F. and Pawlby, S. (1977), 'Individual differences in mothering behaviour: a combined epidemiological and observational approach', in Graham, P. J. (ed.), *Epidemiological Approaches in Child Psychiatry*, London, Academic Press.

World Health Organisation (1978), *Mental Disorders: Glossary and Guide to Their Classification in Accordance with the Ninth Revision of the International Classification of Diseases*, Geneva, WHO.

World Health Organisation (1984), *Health Promotion: A Discussion Document on the Concept and Principles*, Copenhagen, WHO Regional Office for Europe.

Wrede, G., Byring, R., Enberg, S., Huttunen, M., Mednick, S. A. and Nilsson, C. G. (1981), 'A longitudinal study of a risk group in Finland', in Mednick, S. A. and Baert, A. E. (eds), *Prospective Longitudinal Research: An Empirical Basis for the Primary Prevention of Psychosocial Disorders*, Oxford, Oxford University Press.

Author Index

Subject Index

273